FORAGING GUIDE

Identifying and Locating Regional Edible Wild Plants and Mushrooms

MONA GREENY

Table of Contents

Introduction 1

Chapter 1: Forage 5

    Categories of Foraging... 8

    15 Commonly Asked Questions on Foraging........................... 14

Chapter 2: Mushrooms 20

    History of Edible and Non-Edible Mushrooms 20

    Discovery of Mushrooms... 23

    History of Cultivation of Mushrooms 26

    History of Cultivation of Some Specific Species 28

Chapter 3: Mushroom Foraging....................................36

    How to Identify Mushrooms 36

    The Correct Process of Mushroom Identification 37

    Tips to Identify Poisonous Mushrooms............................. 39

    Mushroom Cultivation.. 40

    Essentials of Mushroom Cultivation................................ 40

    6 Critical Steps in Mushroom Cultivation................................ 42

    Species Selection 44

    Key Species and the Cultivation Methods........................... 45

    Assets Required for Mushroom Cultivation 50

Nutritional Values of Mushrooms 51

Mushroom Allergies and Intolerance 53

Symptoms of Allergic Reaction to Mushroom 53

Mushroom Intolerance Remedy 54

Chapter 4: Harvesting and Storage Tips for Mushrooms 55

When to Harvest Mushrooms 56

How to Harvest Mushrooms: Cutting or Picking 56

How to Pick or Cut Mushrooms 57

How to Store Mushrooms 58

Chapter 5: Wild Plants 62

Where Can Wild Plants Be Found? 63

Uses of Wild Plants 64

Environmental Value of Wild Plants 67

Chapter 6: 50 Edible Wide Plants in North America 68

Chickweed 68

Fireweed 70

Wood Sorrels 72

Mustard Greens 74

Wild Black Cherries 76

Alfalfa 78

Dandelions 80

Curly Dock 82

Chicory 83

Creeping Charlie 85

Harebell 86

Broadleaf Plantain 88

Pineapple Weed 89

Mallow 90

Coneflower 92

Elderberry 93

Meadowsweet 94

Pepper Grass... 96

Field Pennycress 97

Purple Deadnettle 98

Forget Me Not 100

Mullein... 101

Bull Thistle 103

Kudzu 104

Pickerelweed 105

Red Clover.. 107

Partridgeberry 108

Sheep Sorrel.. 109

Shepherds Purse 111

Sunflower... 113

Spring Beauty... 114

Tea Plant 116

Toothwort.. 118

Teasel.. 120

Wild Grape Vines 122

Wild Bee Balm 124

Vervain Mallow.. 125

Prickly Pear Cactus.. 126

Herb Robert 128

Mayapple 129

Joe Pye Weed 131

Knapweed 132

Wild Leek 134

Cleavers 135

Cattail.. 137

Blue Vervain.. 138

Common Yarrow... 140

Common Sow Thistle... 141

Coltsfoot 143

Fern Leaf Yarrow.. 144

Final Words... 145

Chapter 7: Harvesting and Storage Tips for Wild Edible Plants. 147

Tips for Harvesting Wild plants 148

Tips for Storing Wild Plants 151

Final Words... 152

Chapter 8: Tips on Foraging 153

General Tips for Foraging 153

Tips to Test Plant Edibility 155

Tips To Consider During Foraging............................... 158

Tips for Forage Clothing.. 160

Additional Tips for Foraging during Hiking Activities 160

Chapter 9: Environmental Benefits and Hazards of Foraging ... 162

    Benefits of Foraging on the Environment 164

    Hazards of Foraging on the Environment.............................. 168

    Final Words... 172

Chapter 10: Essential Tools for Foraging 173

    15 Essential Tools for Foraging... 173

Chapter 11: Foraging Societies: What You Need to Know........ 181

    General Attributes of Foraging Societies............................... 182

    Types of Foraging Societies 184

Conclusion 187

Introduction

B ob was a simple man. He went hiking one day and got lost in the mountains. He had gone alone in the early morning.

His mind had wandered off for a second. Now, he was lost without any idea of where he was in the forest.

To make the matter worse, Bob had not taken any food with him that morning, only a bottle of water. He didn't have a compass on him. The only thing he has was a small Army knife that he always kept on him.

Do you think that he will suffer from hunger? Well, you are wrong if you think he will.

Bob had learned the art of foraging. He knew which plants or mushrooms he could eat to stay refreshed while in the wild.

He put that knowledge to use and was able to survive despite the tough situation. He might even tell you that he enjoyed his time in the mountain forest.

You don't want to wait until you are in a situation like Bob's before you learn about foraging.

The fact is that more and more people are going back to the primitive ways of the hunters-gatherers era. You cannot blame them. If you knew the benefits of foraging, you would be jumping on the lifestyle too.

Are you thinking about what you can gain from looking for food in the wild? The truth is there are a lot of things that you can achieve.

Foraging for food helps you to live a healthier life. The diet of fresh raw food that grows without the addition of chemicals enables you to build a more robust immune system. The food has not been processed in any way that will be harmful to your health.

Some of the things you get to eat when you forage include fruits, edible wild plants, fungi, nuts, and so on. This food can be eaten raw or cooked. Many, if not all, of these meals have more nutrients than food we eat in our daily diets.

Foragers also talk about the medicinal benefits that they get from their forages. There are lots of medicinal plants that this group of people uses instead of conventional drugs. One of the advantages of doing this is the inexistence of side effects from these plants, unlike the traditional medicines that people use.

Do you want to get in some exercise without actually going to a gym? It would be best if you considered a lifestyle of foraging. The time you will spend walking, bending, and searching for forage will help you get some exercise in, giving you a healthier body.

More than the physical benefits, you also get the psychological benefit of feeling connected to the earth. Nature is an essential part of our life, and reconnecting with the universe will help you feel at peace.

Now, you know some of the benefits you can gain from becoming a forager.

Are you eager to get started? Don't rush!

One thing you need to know about foraging is that not all wild plants are edible. Some of these plants are downright poisonous and can kill within minutes.

You don't have to become discouraged by this fact. You can learn how to locate and identify which plant or mushroom is edible and what is not.

Are you wondering how you can get to know this information? Well, that is the aim of this book - to help you locate and identify edible wild plants and mushrooms in your region.

One of the essential tips to note when you want to forage is not to pick up plants that you don't recognize. More times than not, these plants will turn out to be harmful to your health. Even if they are not, since you don't recognize it, there is no way to know for sure.

So, it is best to stay away from these plants.

If you go foraging in a group and someone in your group recognizes the plant as edible, you can still take this plant. However, ensure that the person knows for sure.

There is also an old saying that warns you to leave plants with clusters of three leaves like poison ivy. Plants that have a milky sap can also be dangerous to eat or even touch.

There is a lot that you need to know before you set out to foraging.

However, you don't have to become overwhelmed.

In this book, you would learn all that you need to locate and identify edible wild plants and mushrooms in your environment.

It is time to say yes to a better life by foraging, and our guide will help you concerning all things foraging.

Enjoy your reading!

Chapter 1

Forage

What Does Foraging Entail?

Forage is the activity of getting food from the natural environment. Foraging involves getting edible fruits, birds, insects, and animals from the wild. It also has to do with gathering birds and insects. Foragers also scavenge animals killed by predators.

For some people, foraging for food while hiking or mountaineering is a hobby. They have goods packed, but foraging just completes the whole outing. Although in some situations, it becomes necessary, not just a hobby.

Beyond foraging for food while wildcrafting, this activity has been done by humans for a long time. It is one of the oldest means of survival humans engaged in for food.

In earlier times, some societies based their survival entirely on foraging. Most of these societies were living in desert and forest areas. Planting is not the norm in the places because the plants wouldn't grow.

Some foragers in time past also lived in fertile areas in temperate zones. Some of these areas were river valleys. After some years, these areas became farmlands.

Most people who live their lives as scavengers have dogs. They do not cultivate crops and do not rear animals. Their dogs contribute a lot to their livelihood. They act as pets for the foragers, providing comfort and companionship. The dogs help them in hunting.

When they are out scavenging, the dogs help too, finding sources of food and, sadly, when there is no food, or there is a famine, some scavengers will even eat their dogs.

A society of foragers are people who have been in the game for years. Since it is their primary source of living, they assign roles. The men would hunt for animals. They would also scavenge animals killed by other predators. The women usually picked plants.

There are also activities performed by anyone, gender notwithstanding.

In these instances, the gender lines blur out. Anyone can do about any part of the job. Activities like firewood gathering are the work of anyone. Women and men also hunt for small animals and gather insects.

Some foraging societies are given to relocating rapidly. Their settlement is determined by the availability of food in the area. As a result, they do not establish permanent structures for living.

Sometimes, their movement is determined by the season of crop yield.

Animals forage like humans. However, human foraging is more advanced and strategic. Humans are of a higher class than animals and are enlightened. The knowledge man has helped him in feeding and results in better ways of foraging.

Foraging is an activity that has been with man from time immemorial. Humans have always lived their lives as foragers. From generation to generation, humans have always depended on the earth for sustenance.

Foraging as a method of survival among humans is not new. It is a practice that has spanned about 200,000 years. As time went on, acquired knowledge and technological advancements have birthed new means of survival.

Today, we have supermarkets, stores, restaurants, and even online platforms. These developments have reduced the rate of foraging.

That is not to say that foraging is dying off. It is a practice that is still much with us. Hikers, mountaineers, and tourists do go for foraging. However, there are different categories. We gave explained these categories below.

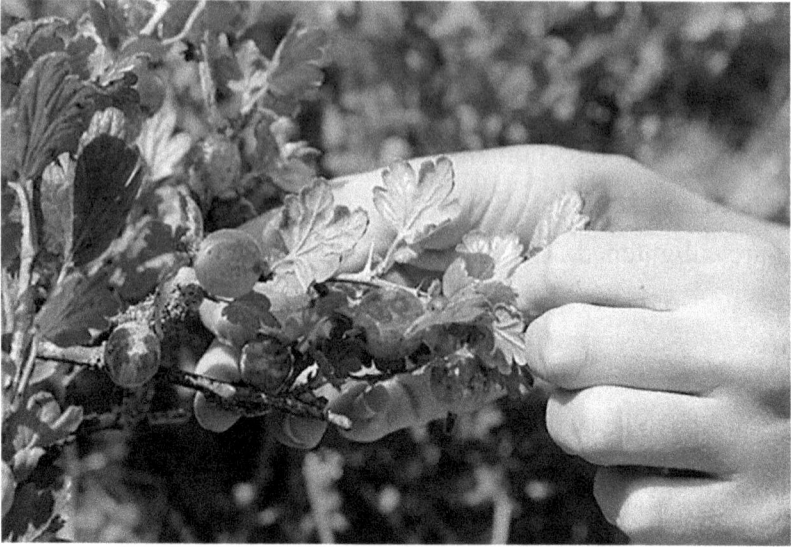

Categories of Foraging

There are different categories of foraging. People go about this exercise in different ways.

Some focus their hunt on aquatic mammals and fishes. This subsistence pattern is referred to as aquatic foraging.

There is equestrian foraging that has to do with hunting game animals with horses.

There are pedestrian foragers who gather foods on foot. Other categories include individual foragers and group foragers.

While some people engage in individual foraging, others forage in groups. Some foragers engage in mushroom hunting and gleaning.

1. Gleaning

Gleaning is a method of foraging that relies on leftovers from farms. When farmers harvest their crops for commercial purposes, there are usually leftovers. Foragers glean the plants for food.

Gleaning also occurs in fields that are harvested. These fields are left to grow because there is no commercial gain from collecting them.

In some parts of Europe like France and England, gleaning is considered the right of poor people. As a result, it was supported by law for peasants to glean from farms and harvested fields.

In the 18th century, England had a law that permitted people without lands to glean. It was their legal right. These landless residents were also referred to as cottagers. However, this constitutional right ended in 1788.

The advantage of this kind of foraging is that harvesting poisonous plants are low, if not non-existent. Since the plants were planning ted by farmers, there is the assurance that the crops are edible.

Foragers are at an advantage with this method of foraging because they are certain of the plants' freshness. Since farmers tended the farms, the crops are most certainly nutritious and fresh.

The advantage is bidirectional. The farmers also benefit from this method. After harvesting, there is the possibility that some crops will be left behind. Foragers save these crops from wasting by harvesting them.

2. Mushroom Hunting

Mushroom hunting is a specialized system of foraging. Foragers who engage in this pattern focus specifically on harvesting mushrooms for food. Some hikers and mountaineers focus their foraging on mushrooms only.

This category of foraging is also called shrooming, mushroom foraging, or mushroom picking. It is a common practice in Korea, Europe, Japan, etc.

Mushroom foragers collect different species of edible mushrooms.

Mushroom hunting is a worthwhile exercise. Aside from mushrooms making good food, they have other benefits.

Collecting mushrooms calls for caution. There are poisonous species that are anything but edible. If you are not sure which is edible or poison, avoid them altogether.

If doing away with mushrooms is a hard decision to make, use a guide. If mushrooming is part of your wildcrafting schedule, use a tour guide. This e-book provides a great guide.

3. Group Foraging

Group foraging involves more than one person. Some families or groups of friends can forage together. A group of hikers or mountaineers can decide to hunt together.

Group foraging is advantageous.

Several hands are working at the same time. A group of foragers can overcome challenges better than an individual. They can pool resources and experiences together and gather more food.

4. Individual Foraging

Unlike group foragers, the individual foragers gather foods alone.

Without a team, he or she hunts for food with his or her skills. A hiker can decide to go foraging without other hikers.

One advantage of this method is that the individual gets to keep the food alone. Whatever quantity is bagged belongs to the individual.

However, the number of foods gathered may not be much. Also, the forager may need friends who have better results, and add to his or her skills and level of expertise. If you choose to go with this pattern, it is not a bad idea.

Since it is a one-person team, you should give ample thought to packing for your journey. Take essential tools that will aid your exercise. If there's any challenge, you should have enough information and tools to tackle it.

5. Equestrian Foraging

Equestrian foraging is a specialized subsistence pattern. It is a dedicated gathering that is focused on specific species.

Equestrian foragers hunt for animals using horses. This type of foraging earned its name "equestrian," which is derived from "Equus," meaning horse in Latin.

Foragers of this sort are found in Southern Argentina, North America, and even South America. This kind of foraging prospers on horse breeding and horse riding skill.

The advantages of equestrian foraging are numerous. For one, it yields a large output. Since the attention is focused on a limited specie, hunting them becomes more efficient. The foragers get to be experts on harvesting these foods. Their catch is usually significant. Food supplies are more.

This method of foraging also has its downsides. Since it is a subsistence pattern that is focused on a limited range of species, it does not allow for much diversity. The food garnered and eaten is limited to the catch made.

Another disadvantage is that consistency of the food is not guaranteed. A catastrophic event like earthquake or fire can result in the animals the foragers hunt being wiped out. An epidemic outbreak can also affect animals.

When events like these occur, and it affects the animals, the foragers specialize in hunting. It can leave them hungry. It is an uncertain way to live life.

6. Aquatic Foraging

Like equestrian foraging, aquatic foraging focuses on specific specie. However, there are differences between them. While equestrian foragers focus their catch on large game animals, aquatic foragers focused on marine animals and fishes.

This foraging pattern earned its name from the Latin word "aqua," which means "water." Aquatic foragers are common in the US, Canada, British Columbia, and other places. The Haida in Queen Charlotte Island forages aquatic foods a lot.

Aquatic foragers usually forage for seaweeds, sea cucumbers, otters, crabs, sea lions, salmon, and other seafood.

The advantage of this foraging system lies in its reliability. Foragers are sure to get food whenever they go foraging. Foragers along coastal areas and rivers are at an advantage. Hikers and mountaineers are confident of making good catches.

7. Pedestrian Foraging

Pedestrian foraging is a standard method of gathering food. This category of foraging is highly mobile. Some foragers who engage in this pattern depend on it as a source of livelihood.

They move from place to place and have temporary settlements. They follow migrating herds and regionally available plants in seasons. The !Kung San or the Zhu|õasi who live in the Kalahari desert is known for pedestrian foraging.

Hikers and mountaineers engage in this method often. While touring an area, they can forage for food in fields around them. Mountaineers can gather nourishment from the lands around the mountains.

The merits of this foraging pattern are that it offers a diversity of harvests. There is the assurance of a continuous food supply. It is sustainable in the long run.

15 Commonly Asked Questions on Foraging

It is the norm to have some questions when venturing into a new path. For anyone considering foraging, some questions will pop up in your mind. Some seasoned foragers might also have one or two inquiries as well.

Here are 15 commonly asked questions on forage.

1. Why Should I Forage?

This question is excellent, but you should be able to ask yourself and provide the answer to it. Before setting out, be sure you have the right reason. It will keep you motivated when you have challenges. Also, it will determine how you go about your business.

People forage for different reasons. Some foragers aim to foster a connection with nature. Some people look for food because they want to have fun harvesting wild plants. You should know why you forage.

2. What are the Benefits of Foraging?

Most people who are considering forage ask this question. Perhaps, you know people who forage and are thinking of joining them, but you want to be sure of what you're going into.

Foraging is fun, especially when you're going with a group. But beyond the fun, there are responsibilities attached. You may want to know the benefits before giving it a go.

It is essential to know the benefits of foraging because it will propel you forward. Also, it will give you a sense of achievement in the long run.

3. How Do I Prepare for Foraging?

Before you pack your bags and hit the road, you have to prepare well. You need to put thought into the whole backpacking thing. You should think the entire process through down to foraging. It is wise to consult foraging books and articles.

You can also ask questions. Perhaps, you know someone who has walked the path you plan to walk, tap from their wealth of knowledge. There are guides on different categories of forage.

4. What Should I Know about My Location?

If you are a hiker or mountaineer, you may do more than just climbing mountains or hiking. You may want to go foraging. If this is your decision, be sure to know some basics about the place.

Know your location thoroughly or enough to avoid missing your way. Familiarize yourself with the terrain. Know the possible threats to life and possible escape routes.

Ensure that you do not trespass. If you are not in a public area, tread with caution. Do not violate a private area. Know the law binding in your location and adhere to them.

You do not want your experience to go sour. Use a field guide to be on a safe side. They most likely know what you do not know.

5. What is the Best Time of Year to Forage?

After picking your location, you have to do your homework. Know about it in total. However, it does not end there. You have to know the best time of year to visit there.

If this is your next step in preparing to forage, then you are right on track. You can find a mix of things around the year, but there are specific seasons for different plants.

July to mid-October is the season for mushrooms. However, you can get more varieties of mushrooms in September. April is the time for a wide range of plants.

6. What Safety Measures Should I Take?

Safety is everything. You have to observe safety measures to have a smooth experience backpacking and foraging. A location expert comes handy here.

If you have underlying health issues, sort yourself out before wildcrafting. If you must set out, then take your necessities along like drugs.

Take the right tools for foraging. Mind the plants you eat; not all wild plants are edible.

If it is your first time, go with a group. You can venture out on your own when you have gained some experience.

7. What's the Best Place to Forage for Plants?

Foraging is a fun way of getting edibles. However, you want to be sure where to get enough catch for your satisfaction.

The basics are that you can forage anywhere you go. If you're hiking, mountaineering, or otherwise, you are likely to get edible wild plants. These plants can be found in fields, forests, and so on.

8. How Do I Book with a Good Forage Company?

Where you book, your tour will determine the experience you have. The forage company you work with matters a lot. Get good companies with an outstanding reputation.

Get friends and family members who have gone foraging before to recommend agencies for you. Some touring companies are known for accidents and unfavorable customer services.

Before you strike a deal with the company, know their policies and rules to see if it suits you. Some companies have specific months they are open for work. Some of these companies are closed sometimes because of the weather condition.

9. What Tools Do I Need to Forage?

The tools required for foraging differ with the category of foraging.

The environment you will forage in also matters. Perhaps when you go hiking or mountain climbing, you may want to forage for food.

Before setting out, you should determine if you will forage and how you will go about it. This decision will determine the tools to use.

Another consideration is if you will forage alone or with a group. If you are going with a group, there is a chance of having all the necessary tools. If everyone pool resources together, they can come up with practical tools for hunting.

10. How Do I Know Edibles Plants to Forage?

While foraging is a great way to feed and have fun, you also have to be careful. Not all wild plants are edible. Even some mushrooms are poisonous.

It is advisable to know what plants are generally obtainable in your location. You also need to know the wild plants in season. Double-check plants with white or discoloring sap and determine their edibility. They most likely are not safe.

If you don't know the specie of an edible plant, it is better to avoid that plant entirely. The rule is to avoid eating anything you are not 100% certain is edible. If you are familiar with any plant, stick to it.

11. How Do I Avoid Deadly Plants?

Use a field guide! Some edible plants are similar to poisonous ones. Some plants have edible and toxic parts. If in doubt, don't risk it.

12. How Do I Harvest Wild Plants and Mushrooms?

You should know how to gather plants without killing them off while foraging. It is advisable to use a knife or shear. Some plants should not be uprooted to preserve their kinds.

13. How Do I Handle My Harvest or Catch?

It is reasonable to ask how to handle your catch or harvest. It is one thing to forage; it is another to preserve your catch well. The kind of food you plan to get will determine the way you will keep it.

The essential thing is to know how to transport and clean your harvest. You also need to know how to skin your catch before consumption.

14. Is It Legal to Forage in My Chosen Area?

Before you go foraging, it is essential to know the legal provisions in your area. Legality varies among regions and even countries. In some places, foraging could be considered theft. The 1968 Theft Act in the UK kicks against selling produce from forage.

If you are foraging in an uninhabited area, be careful not to infringe on private property.

If you must forage in a garden or farm, take proper permission from the owner. If you are not granted access, anything you take will be considered theft.

You may strike a deal with the landowner on splitting your catch or harvest.

15. Should I Join A Foraging Society?

Foraging societies consist of people who live their lives foraging. They go from place to place, gathering foods and animals. It may be your desire to go with these societies once in a while.

Chapter 2

Mushrooms

M ushrooms are a particular type of fungus that grow like plants. Often, they are confused as vegetables. While this assumption isn't entirely wrong, they are best described as fungus.

The most widely consumed species is the button mushroom (Agaricus bisporus). It has claims to history as it is the first species cultivated in the western world. As of today, it accounts for over 40% of the world's cultivation of mushrooms.

At some point, you might have wondered, "who discovered these mushrooms?". Probably you were awed by their delicious taste in a soup. Maybe, you are fascinated by their beauty. Either way, you probably did not get an answer.

In this chapter, you will get to find out the history of mushrooms.

History of Edible and Non-Edible Mushrooms

Mushrooms have been here for a while, no doubt. Over the years of their existence, man has used them extensively for different purposes. The delicious delicacies that come from them are probably the most common of all uses.

Delicious, deadly, intoxicating is a few words to describe mushrooms. Some might even go further to add magical. Throughout history, mushrooms have meant different things to different people.

According to food historians, humans have long consumed mushrooms. From prehistoric times, man has been eating these fungi, both edible and poisonous. Historians believe that man stumbled upon it during the hunting and foraging period.

It is no doubt that our perception of them dramatically differs from the times of old. In the past, hunters gathered them, and eating them was something of a trial and error exercise. In most of those cases, there were no happy endings.

At the time, their method of cultivation wasn't known. Unlike natural plants, they couldn't be grown at home. Therefore, they had to be collected when needed. Even until now, the cultivation of many species is still unknown.

The fatal end from the consumption of some mushrooms made some people detest it. Even though some edible species were known, some people stay away outrightly. It led to the classification of people as mycophile and mycophobes.

Mycophiles are people who enjoy eating mushrooms. Mycophobes, on the other hand, are those who fear mushrooms. Generally, people from the eastern part of the world were mostly Mycophiles. People from western cultures were mostly Mycophobes.

A French philosopher once said mushrooms changed the destiny of Europe. Many historians believed he meant the Austrian succession war. The war was said to have followed the demise of Holy Roman Emperor King Charles VI.

Many people claim that the king's death was as a result of consuming amanita mushrooms. Amanita, also called death cap, is very deadly.

Several notable people have died by ingesting poisonous mushrooms. The physicist who invented the Fahrenheit lost his parents to mushroom poisoning in 1701.

Johann Schobert, a French composer, alongside his wife and daughter, died in 1767. This happening was after he had insisted that a poisonous mushroom was edible.

On the other side of the world, however, they were embraced. The Chinese and the Japanese, in particular, had consumed them for their health benefits.

Until recently in history, these fungi plants never really had names. This omission was because they were considered mysterious in many cultures. For instance, in ancient Egypt, mushrooms were thought to have immortality powers. For that reason, only Pharaohs had the right to eat them.

Similarly, in ancient Rome, it was only eaten by the wealthy families. Historians claim that Caesars employed tasters in a bid to prevent poisoning. The tasters were to vet the food to ensure it was safe enough for eating.

The Greeks were also known to have imported it from Libya. They were then sold along the south of Europe.

Discovery of Mushrooms

It is difficult to say who, where, and when mushrooms were discovered. However, archeological findings have proven that mushrooms were used in prehistoric times.

For example, in the Tassili caves of Algeria, there are rock paintings of mushrooms. These paintings are believed to have existed for about 7,000 years. Similarly, in Spain, rock paintings dating back to 6,000 years have also be found. Evidence, in general, point to 9000BC as the period of its first use.

The first record of them in Europe is traced back to the Greek philosopher Hippocrates. Hippocrates is said to have first documented their medicinal use. This document belonging to Hippocrates is believed to have been written around 400BC.

The name 'mushroom' is from two French words. The two words mean Fungi and mold. Although this name only came to be in recent times.

In Northern Africa, the Psilocybe mairei and the Psilocybe hispanica are notably depicted in most of the rock paintings. These two species are worthy of note because of their hallucinogenic properties. According to some experts, these species were used for their medicinal benefits.

The documentations on its consumption in Egypt date back as far as 4500BC. Many ancient wall arts depicting plants feature mushrooms. Also, pillars were molded in the shape of mushrooms. Many of which can still be found today.

Many old texts from ancient Egypt also talk about mushrooms, mainly, 'the Egyptian Book of the Dead.' In the book, the author is quoted as saying, 'it's the food of the gods.'

Also, an ancient poem attributed to Egypt reads as follows:

> "Without leaves, without buds, without flowers: yet they from fruit; as a food, as a tonic, as medicine: the entire creation is precious."

In ancient China, Greece, and Mexico, mushrooms were used for ritual purposes. Even in Spain, the rock paintings have some depictions of ritual purposes of mushrooms.

Around that time, there were lots of myths attached to mushrooms. Some believed it could unlock superhuman abilities. Others thought it could connect humans with the dead, and others thought it could direct ones' soul. Some people also believe it can lead one to the gods.

It would interest you to know that even until now, many of these beliefs still exist. For instance, Mexicans still use mushrooms with hallucinogenic materials for rituals. In such ceremonies, participants are believed to 'see' the gods.

The use of hallucinogenic mushrooms in the Mesoamerican region reduced around the 1500s. Writings from priests that date back to the 1500s described the use and effects of the mushrooms extensively.

The Catholic missionaries promptly discouraged its use. Subsequently, people were killed for using the mushrooms in the region. The use was restricted to ritual ceremonies. Even at that, consumption continued mostly privately.

In 1916, these hallucinogenic mushrooms, also called magic mushrooms, attracted the attention of modern medicine. Dr. William Safford disproved their existence after going through some Spanish records. According to him, nothing in the world could give such intoxicating effects.

In subsequent years in the 1930s, scientists trooped into Central America. Their mission was to see for themselves if such mushrooms existed or Safford's claims were valid.

It wasn't until 1955 that R. Gordon Wasson found the mushrooms. He took part in a ritual ceremony in Mexico. After that, he, alongside his wife and daughter, took part in the rituals. In 1957, he published an article, "Seeking the Magic Mushroom."

In 1962, Albert Hoffman discovered that psilocybin and psilocin were responsible for the mushroom's hallucinogenic properties. In 1968, after about 11 years of use, the drug was banned in the US.

History of Cultivation of Mushrooms

There are some controversies as to how the cultivation of mushrooms started. Western cultures claim that it began in 1650. You might find that the dates differ from different texts. However, we are sure that it began around the mid-1600s.

Contrary to this narrative, evidence proves that the cultivation of mushrooms started in China and Japan as far back as 200 BC. Even though it is speculative, some experts claim it could be older than that.

Historians claim that Auricularia polytricha was the first species to be grown in ancient China. Auricularia polytricha is also known as ear fungus. The mushroom was cultivated for its many medicinal properties.

In western culture, cultivation started in France. The cultivation, which started by accident, is attributed to a melon grower that stayed around Paris. Button mushroom or shop mushroom (Agaricus bisporus) was the species that was first cultivated.

History has it that the melon grower found the mushroom growing on manure. After this discovery, he decided to grow them commercially. Fortunately, his attempt at commercialization was very successful.

Since it was successful, he sold them to restaurants around Paris. The mushroom got its nickname 'Parisian mushroom' around this period. This form of cultivation continued for a long time. Even till date, some farmers still cultivate Agaricus bisporus using this method.

Some years later, a gardener in France, named Chambry discovered a better way to grow them. Some controversies, however, exist around this fact. While some texts would claim they are the same persons, some say they are two different people.

He found out that mushrooms were better grown in caves than in the open field. This advantage was due to the cold and moist environment that the caves provided.

This discovery changed the dynamics of mushroom cultivation in France. From then onwards, people started to grow them in large quantities. To date, many of the caves in France are used for this purpose.

It took until the 1800s nearly 200 years later, before mushrooms were accepted in Europe. In America, it was first accepted as a condiment. As time went on, mushrooms became a part of Native American meals.

Many historians have claimed that the French introduced mushrooms to England and America. Within a short period, Americans adopted it well. Foraging clubs began to develop across the country. Their main aim was the collection and identification of the edible species.

Cultivation first started in America with farmers using dark areas under greenhouse benches. In 1894, a building was constructed for the sole purpose of growing mushrooms. It was the first of its kind in the world at the time. The building is located in Pennsylvania to date.

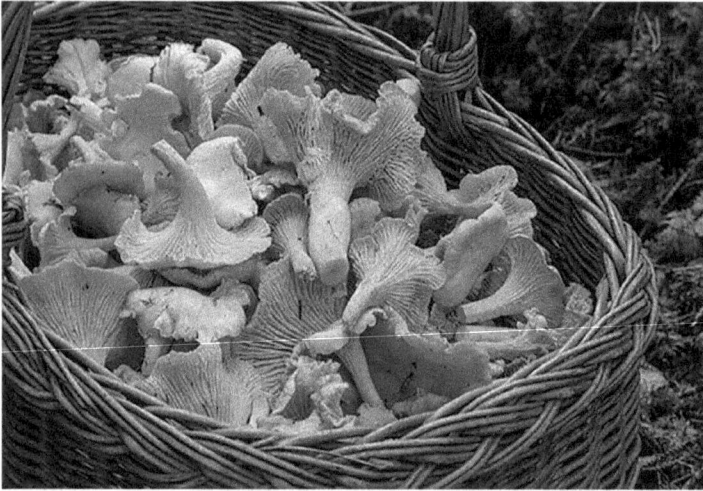

History of Cultivation of Some Specific Species

Since the inception of cultivating mushrooms, there has been a lot of improvements. Cultivation methods for different species are emerging daily. However, many of those inventions came on recently with the rise of technological advancement.

However, the knowledge we have so far about them is still limited compared to the number of edible species that we have. Humans can cultivate only a few species as of today.

Here are a few of those species and how their cultivation methods were discovered.

1. Button Mushroom (Agaricus bisporus)

Many people are familiar with this species of mushroom. It is by far the most popular of all.

Also called 'shop mushroom,' it is the most cultivated species in the world. Until around the end of the 1970s, it was the only cultivated species in the world.

Cultivation of this mushroom started in the 1600s. As stated earlier, it began in France. They were grown in the open fields for about 160 years. Sometime afterward, it was discovered that the mushrooms grow from their spawn or mycelium.

This method was somewhat similar to growing plants from seeds. Later on, in France as well, it was discovered that light was not needed for their growth.

This knowledge led to a shift from open field cultivation to cultivation in caves. In 1910, the French started growing this species in conventional houses. However, to date, caves are still preferred for cultivation.

During the 1800s, the cultivation of Agaricus bisporus spread to England. In 1856, it was introduced to the US from England. Initially, the mycelia had to be imported from England to the US. These efforts proved abortive as many of the spawns were damaged on arrival to the US.

There had to be indigenous spawns in the US to mitigate this loss. In 1903, the scientists of the US Department of Agriculture successfully developed one.

2. Ear Fungus (Auricularia polytricha and Auricularia auricula)

These two species are classified under the jelly fungi. They are the most popular of all edibles in this category. Auricularia polytricha is mainly found around warmer tropical environments. Auricularia auricula, on the other hand, is located in temperate climates.

They might be the oldest known cultivated mushrooms in the world. Their cultivation started long ago in China and Japan between 200 and 300BC.

The species are saprophytic. This term means that they feed on dead decaying things. Therefore, in ancient China, they were grown on the trunks of dead trees. To date, it is still very much the practice.

They are named after the distinct ear shape they have.

3. Oyster Mushrooms

Mushrooms belonging to the genus Pleurotus fall under this category. Over the years, a good number of the mushrooms in this category have been cultivated.

Before their cultivation, they were collected mainly in North America and Europe. They were a popular species amongst foragers at the time. Even now, they remain popular options.

Until the beginning of the 20th century, nothing was known about their cultivation. Around the 1970s, a method or cultivation for Pleurotus ostreatus was first described.

The method involved growing the species on dead logs of wood. The system wasn't much of an invention. It was more of modification as it had been used in China over 800 years before then.

The ancient Chinese people had used the method to grow other species. The technique was, however, not so efficient. The logs sometimes got infected and produced other species that weren't intended. This happening led to several modifications of the method to suit its production.

4. Truffles (Tuber melanosporum)

Truffles are a particular type of mushrooms. They are highly-priced and much sought after. As of 2011, a pound of Black Truffle (Tuber melanosporum), cost about 1000 dollars. The white type (Tuber magnatum) was sold between 1000 dollars and 2200 dollars in 2001.

Though the genus Tuber contains very many species, only a few of them are edible. The gathering of this species date back to 1600BC. Many scientists at the time developed theories about their nature and origin.

Theophrastus is said to be the first person to come up with a hypothesis about them. In his theory, he described them as plants.

He also went further to say their growth was a result of thunderstorms and rain.

This misconception went on for years. This concept was accepted because truffles grow underground.

In 1885, a plant pathologist from Germany developed a different hypothesis. He described the true nature of truffles. He also went further to explain that they had a sort of symbiotic relationship with tree roots.

His theories were rejected and then later accepted in the early parts of the 20th century. Even afterward, many still believe truffles are products of trees where they are found. A lot of mysteries still surround the complicated relationship between truffles and tree roots.

Many theories that abound about the relationship are mostly speculative. To date, a lot of shadows still abound around its production. There are no known methods of cultivation yet.

Due to these mysteries, the consumption of truffles has mostly depended on natural collection. Around the time of the world wars, there was a drop in the demand for truffles. This drop in demand resulted in a sharp decline in prices across the globe.

The once valued truffles became useless. Farmers had to pull the trees where they were growing. They did this to give way for more profitable crops.

The end of world war II witnessed a sudden surge in demand for truffles. With little supply, the prices surged as well. There was a severe need to balance the growing demand and the thinning supply of truffles.

In 1972, two scientists, Delmas and Grente, proposed a means of propagation. They suggested that trees should be inoculated with the Truffle mycelia.

Five years later, the first trial was carried out in Europe. A vast expanse of land was used, which contained Hazel trees and Oak plantations. The trees were then inoculated with Truffle mycelia. The first harvest took about ten years, and it was successful.

The method was very productive, as well as sustainable. The trees continued to produce Truffles as long as the trees stayed alive.

5. Morels Genus Morchella

Just like Truffles, little is known about the cultivation of morels. Like truffles too, they are expensive. However, unlike truffles, all species of morels are edible.

Cultivating morels has been an issue for a long time in history. In France, 1883, morels were reported to have been cultivated in the fields. The report was then followed by a claim

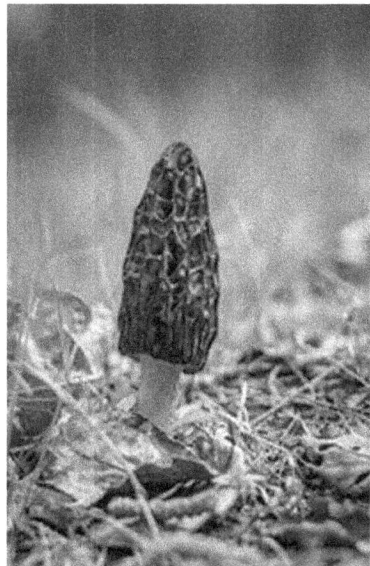

in 1904 by Molliard. He allegedly claimed to have grown morels on compost made from apples. This claim was soon dispelled as it seemed the morels grew naturally.

Scientists have tried to reproduce them in unique environments where they are common. Unfortunately, the experiments failed as morels were not produced.

In the 1950s, morel mycelia were produced. The mycelia were to be used as flavors for cooking. This thinking quickly phased out as people preferred the morels to the mycelia.

In 1982, a method of propagation was developed by Ron Ower in the US. The technique was soon neglected as it was expensive, and it generated very little morels.

Three years later, Ron and Gary Mills improved on the previous method. Although it was better than Ower's approach, the experiment only worked in Michigan. Many variations are available today as regards the cultivation methods. However, no one has been able to develop a profitable practice.

Now, you know that throughout history, mushrooms have been prominent across cultures of the world. In the eastern civilizations of Asia, they were seen as healthy food. In Rome, they were fed to soldiers for strength. Many cultures regarded them as food for the gods.

Mushrooms divided the world into two; the mycophiles and the mycophobes. However, this disparity is fast disappearing. Are you interested in joining the fast-growing group of mycophiles who foraged for mushroom? You will learn all that you need to know from the next chapter. Just keep reading!

Chapter 3

Mushroom Foraging

When some folks go hiking and spot a mushroom in the forest, they simply go in the other direction. When people who hate seeing mushrooms spot one growing on their lawn, they kick it or chemically terminate it.

The dislike these people have for mushrooms is understandable as many mushrooms are poisonous, and only a few are edible. However, if you can give yourself to learning how to identify edible mushrooms, you can begin to enjoy the benefits that mushrooms provide.

How to Identify Mushrooms

Some mushrooms are lovely to eat, many others are toxic, causing severe or temporary discomfort, and most mushrooms are unpalatable or tasteless. The challenge is how to identify the few edible mushrooms.

There are thousands of mushroom species around the world, with some having strange shapes, while some don't look like mushrooms. As you venture further into the mushroom kingdom, you begin to see how the world of mushrooms is complex and intricate.

However, identifying edible mushrooms is not an impossible task. There are processes to follow, as discussed below.

The Correct Process of Mushroom Identification

The mushroom identification process starts with knowing the characteristics of various mushrooms. This stage can come easily if your focus is to identify a few mushrooms.

However, if you want to expand into identifying a wide variety of mushrooms, you will need a mushroom identification book.

There are several mushrooms in the wild that area lookalike of some edible mushrooms, and you can easily mistake them for what they are not. The mushroom identification book serves as your guide to differentiate between the lookalike and the edible mushrooms.

Aside from that, these are four stages to identifying any mushroom;

• Observation

Any mushroom will willingly give its identity away if you know what to look for. What then should you look for in a mushroom?

Begin by looking at its cap. Take note of its length, width, color, and shape.

Also, check under the cap. Note its distinctive features such as color, spacing, strip attachment, etc.

The next thing is to check the stem. Check for striations, stripes, rings, and other identifying features.

Its substrate is also an important thing to check. Where and what is the mushroom growing on?

And lastly, confirm the season of growth. Mushrooms grow at different times in the year. Check to see if it's growing at the right time. If not, it is most likely a lookalike.

• **Examination**

When examining mushrooms, what you do is smell it, feel it, and taste it.

Edible mushrooms have nice smells that can help you identify them. If it doesn't smell great, then it's most likely not an edible mushroom.

It's also important to note how the mushroom feels when you touch it. Edible mushrooms usually feel smooth, fuzzy, slimy, and pleasant to touch.

Lastly, go ahead to taste the mushroom. Cut a portion of it and place it on your tongue then, spit it out. If it tastes bitter, it's an indication to stay away from it. And, don't worry, it won't harm you if you spit it out.

• **Use Key**

At this point, you bring out the mushroom identification book to check the characteristics as described in the book. If it's not what you think it is, it might just be another edible mushroom.

• **Check and Confirm Answers**

Finally, if you have observed, examined, and cross-checked, it is the time to decide based on the characteristics you have found. Note that if it is not 100 percent in agreement with what the features say, stay away from such mushroom.

Tips to Identify Poisonous Mushrooms

There is no single rule that guides the identification of poisonous mushrooms. But, when you come across a mushroom, a few defining characteristics could help you determine if it's toxic or not.

Take note of the following tips to avoid picking mushrooms that may be poisonous by mistake;

- Don't pick mushrooms with white gills

- Avoid mushrooms with a skirt or ring on the stalk

- Avoid mushrooms that have red caps or stalks

These are not definitive as some edible mushrooms can also exhibit some of these characteristics. However, when you notice them, it's a good indication that you need to stay away from such mushrooms.

You may miss out on a tasty mushroom, but you are at least sure that you won't get sick from the consumption of a poisonous mushroom. Note that, for safety reasons, you shouldn't eat any mushroom, if you are not 100 percent sure about its edibility.

Mushroom Cultivation

You love hiking and walking in the woods. But, you don't want to go through the stress of foraging for edible mushrooms every time you want to spice your meal with them. Mushroom cultivation is the answer you seek.

Mushroom cultivation is one sure way to get the type of mushrooms you need either on a small scale or commercial scale. Mushroom foraging is a gamble, especially if you are new to the game. Even experts sometimes make mistakes.

But, when you grow your mushrooms, you can't get it wrong.

Also, those who love a particular type of mushroom may find it difficult to find it in the grocery store. In such a case, growing your mushroom colony is the best solution to the quick access you desire.

With a few tools and the proper growing system, you can have more than enough mushrooms anytime you need them.

Essentials of Mushroom Cultivation

Cultivated mushrooms are edible mushrooms that you grow on decaying organic substances.

You should know the classification of the different mushroom species based on how they tap nutrients to understand the essentials needed for mushroom cultivation. The classifications are;

• Saprobic

A saprobic plant is one that grows on dead organic substances. Saprobic edibles are valued for their food and medicine.

In their cultivated form, they require a constant supply of organic matters suitable to sustain their production. Otherwise, it can be a limiting factor in production.

• Symbiotic

A symbiotic mushroom grows in association with other organisms. They are mostly found in the wild on trees.

The relationship works in that the mushroom helps the tree gather extensive water catchments and help deliver nutrients from the soil that the tree cannot access.

• Parasitic or Pathogenic

Most pathogenic fungi cause diseases to plants. Only a small number of such fungi are edible.

These are the three major classifications of the thousands of mushroom species.

Therefore, mushrooms species are primarily cultivated in two ways:

1. Composted Substrate

Composted substrates are organic matters from substances like rice and wheat straw, hay, corn curb, composted manure, water hyacinth, and several other agricultural by-products including banana leaves and coffee husks.

2. Woody Substrate

This method majorly involves substances such as sawdust, wood logs, or any by-products of wood.

6 Critical Steps in Mushroom Cultivation

The basic concept in mushroom production or cultivation begins with some mushroom spores. These spores grow into mycelium, expanding into massive stored up energy and sufficient mass to support the final phase in the mushroom reproduction cycle.

The formation of mushroom or fruiting bodies is the last phase of the mushroom reproduction cycle. A complete cycle, from start to finish, usually takes between two to three months, depending on the mushroom species.

The vital generic steps in the production process are;

1. Identify and Clean Cultivation Space

You'll need to decide on the room or building to use for cultivation and clean the room. Ensure that you choose a place where you can control the moisture, temperature, and sanitary condition. Those are the conditions that determine the growth of the spores.

2. Growing Medium

There are two primary growing mediums for mushroom cultivation, as stated above. Choose the growing medium you find convenient to work with or that suits the growing environment you have chosen. Then, store the raw ingredients in a clean place and protect it from rain.

3. Pasteurize Medium

You'll need to pasteurize or sterilize the medium and table or bags in which the mushrooms will grow. This sterilization ensures you exclude other fungi from growing on the same platform, thereby competing for nutrients. When the mushroom begins to grow, it colonizes the substance and fights off all competitions.

4. Seeding

When you've done all that, the next step is to seed the bed with spawn.

5. Coordinated Growing Environment

This stage is the most challenging because it is at this point that most of the work is done. You need to maintain optimal moisture, temperature, hygiene, and other conditions that make for the proper growth of mycelium and fruiting. You'll also need to add water to the substrate regularly to raise the moisture content.

6. Harvesting and Recycle

Harvesting is the last stage of the mushroom reproduction process. You process your mushrooms for eating or package for selling at this point. After this, you clean the room and start over again.

Species Selection

Most mushroom species only bear fruits in an environment of about 20 degrees Celsius. Therefore, you will hardly find one growing in a temperate climate. You should stimulate the growing environment temperature to cultivate mushrooms.

Aside from that, the other factors to consider in choosing species to grow to include:

1. Availability of Waste materials for Growing

Not all mushrooms fruit in the same substrate. You should determine the type of substrate you have available before you choose the mushroom species.

2. Condition of the Environment

Different species have environmental conditions in which they thrive. As explained earlier, most mushroom species have difficulty growing in temperate regions. If you reside in a tropical zone, you can only grow varieties that will survive such areas.

3. The Expertise You Have

Some species don't grow easily because of the level of expertise needed to produce them. If you do not know to grow such species and you don't have an expert that you can consult, it's best to start with simpler species like oysters. Shiitake and maitake mushrooms are also a viable option.

4. The Resources You Have

Aside from having enough waste materials needed to support the species you choose, you also need to consider the availability of the resources required to grow such species.

If you'll need to coordinate the environmental temperature for the species to survive, do you have what it takes to achieve that? Also, consider other resources required and judge if you dare to venture into growing such species.

5. Demand in the Market

You might not worry about market demand if you are only growing for personal consumption. On the other hand, if you're growing for commercial use, then you must consider the market demand for such species.

Some people prefer some particular species with an unrepentant bias to some other species. You might need to do a market survey to determine the best mushroom species to grow within your catchment area.

Key Species and the Cultivation Methods

Here are some of the commonly cultivated edible mushroom species accepted globally.

White Button Mushroom (Agaricus Bisporus)

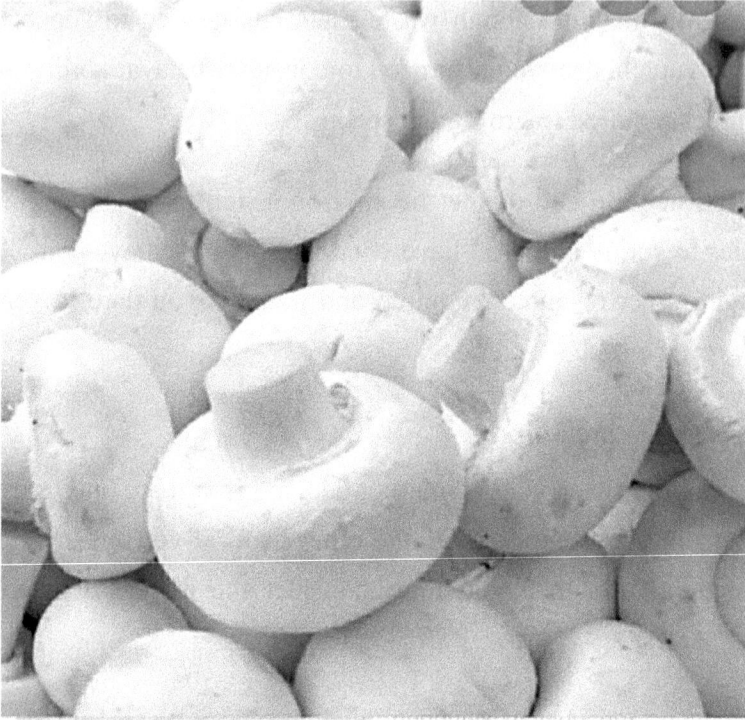

The white button is top on the list of cultivated edible mushrooms by farmers around the world, most grown in temperate regions. You can grow the mushroom in a composted substrate.

You will need higher technology systems because a consistent temperature of 14 to 18 degrees Celsius is required when growing the Agaricus Bisporus. Though it can grow at a higher temperature, it needs to grow in an environment within that temperature to get the best of its fruiting process.

Oyster Mushroom (Pleurotus ostreatus)

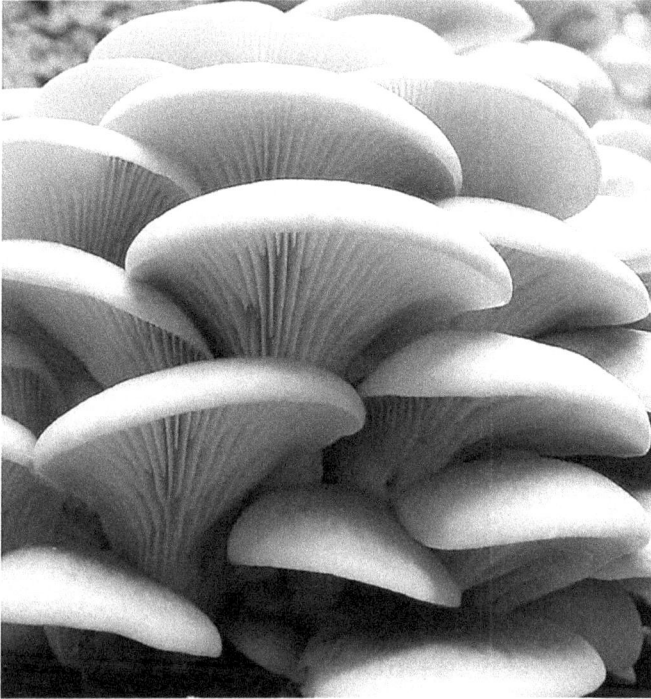

Oyster mushrooms are easier to cultivate compared to other mushroom species. Therefore, they are the best choice for inexperienced mushroom farmers. Besides, their farming process helps utilize farm waste, consequently, becoming an integral part of a sustainable agricultural system.

Cultivators normally grow Oyster on tree logs. People started growing them on sawdust, rice, or wheat straw, and other variety of waste materials having high-cellulose recently. Growing oysters on high-cellulose waste materials reduce its fruiting period to about two months.

The cultivation process involves placing the substrate in a plastic bag, and keeping it in a cool and dark place. As the mycelium grows on the substrate, you should cut an opening in the bag, allowing the fruiting bodies to develop.

Shiitake Mushrooms (Lentinus edodes)

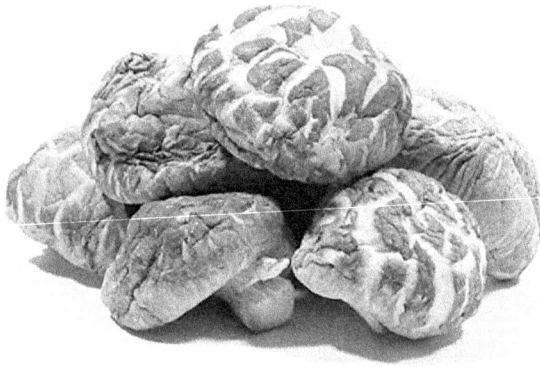

Shiitake mushrooms grow easily and require little resources. You can grow shiitakes, both outdoors and indoors. When outdoors, you can cultivate it on a log, and when indoors, you grow it on sawdust or in bags.

The cultivation system that involves sawdust speeds up the fruiting cycle and increases the returns you get. However, it needs more skillful management than when logs are used.

When you cultivate your mushrooms using logs, the fruiting bodies appear faster based on the diameter of the substrate logs. How long the product will last also depends on how dense the wood is.

Paddy Straw Mushrooms (Volvariella volvacea)

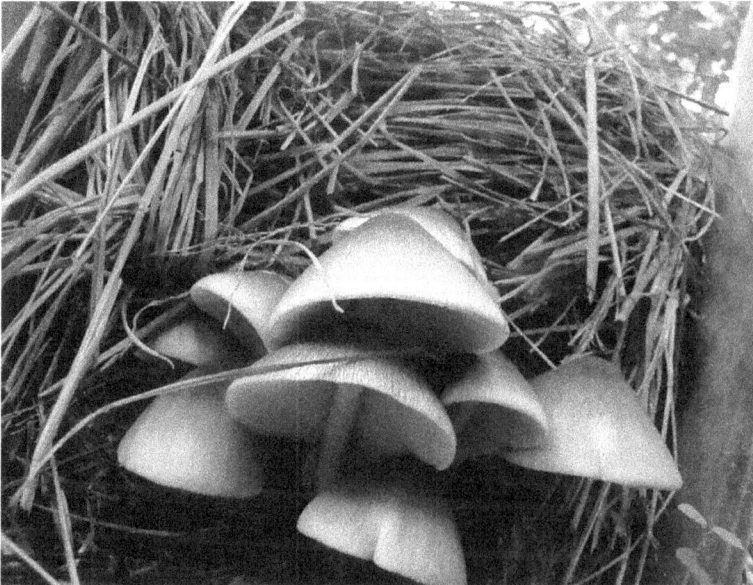

Paddy Straw Mushrooms are cultivated along with rice production. However, you can also grow it on substrates in addition to paddy straw, cotton waste, rice straw, oil palm bunch waste, and dried banana leaves. However, this method yields fewer returns.

In many rural areas, mushroom cultivators just leave thoroughly moistened paddy straw under trees and wait for the mushrooms to grow.

Assets Required for Mushroom Cultivation

Mushroom cultivation demand several activities that people with diverse interests, various needs, and specific capabilities can do. Find the crucial assets you need to cultivate mushrooms below.

1. Natural Assets

Land and climatic conditions play a small role in mushroom cultivation, which makes it possible for farmers with limited area to join in the enterprise. Also, the unpredictable production that plagues the typical farming system does not apply to mushroom cultivation.

Access to sufficient and locally-sourced spore substrate is an essential determinant for the success of mushroom cultivation. How easy is it to get agricultural by-products, logs, or sawdust as the mushroom specie requires, and how cheap is it? You can also get spores from mature fruiting bodies or buy them from local facilities.

2. Human Assets

Human assets mean the skills, knowledge, and ability to work needed to do a line of work. Mushroom cultivation requires little human efforts, and you can operate them as an addition to other tasks.

Because it isn't labor-intensive, people with disabilities can also do mushroom farming and carry out the required tasks. People with mental disabilities can also grow mushrooms because a majority of the tasks involved are repetitive.

3. Physical Assets

The physical equipment needed to grow mushrooms depend on how large the production is. However, many of the physical assets for growing mushrooms are inclusive tools. These items are typical needs such as water, transportation, source of energy, and buildings.

Mushrooms grow best in a cool, enclosed building. In this structure, you can easily maintain the environmental elements such as temperature, humidity, moisture level, and proper ventilation. These conditions allow for proper growth.

4. Financial Assets

The sale of the production determines the financial capacity you need for mushroom cultivation. Since you can grow mushrooms on any scale, the financial commitment to begin a mushroom cultivation system need not be huge. Besides, substrates in the form of agricultural by-products, or logs are often gotten for free.

Compared to other agricultural and horticultural crops, mushroom cultivation systems allow for harvesting after a short time. You can grow mushrooms and harvest them within two to four months. Small scale producers find this an advantage.

Nutritional Values of Mushrooms

Though some mushrooms can be poisonous, we cannot discard the fact that they have nutritional as well as medicinal values. While the nutritional and medicinal values present in mushrooms are different according to the specie, see some of the general benefits below.

1. Nutritional Value

Mushrooms add flavor to food, enhancing the taste of bland foods. They are also a valuable source of food in their own right. Fleshy mushrooms can replace meat and have enough nutrients to compete with several vegetables.

Mushrooms can be added to a meal for a balanced diet, which is of great value, especially to people in developing countries. They are a good source of vitamin B, C, and D, and several other minerals like copper, phosphorus, potassium, and iron.

They also provide carbohydrates and are low in cholesterol, fiber, as well as starch. Furthermore, they are a good source of protein. Mushrooms reportedly contain between 19 to 35 percent of protein, higher than that of kidney beans.

2. Medicinal Value

In addition to the nutritional values, mushrooms have medicinal benefits of polysaccharides, and those are good for boosting your immune system. Now that there's recent promotion of functional foods and focus on other products "that is more than food," mushrooms are a perfect fit into that category.

Mushrooms have routinely been added to Chinese traditional medicines in history. Now, more than six percent of edible mushrooms play a part in many of today's health tonics and herbal formulas.

Mushroom Allergies and Intolerance

Mushroom allergies mistakenly trigger your immune system, thinking the proteins present in mushrooms are dangerous. The immune system creates an influx of histamine, the hormone that protects you from infections and diseases. When it happens, your body reacts funnily, indicating that you're allergic to what you took.

Mushroom intolerance, on the other hand, is more about your genetic coding. It has to do with the difficulty you have in digesting mushrooms. Therefore, you begin to have unpleasant physical reactions to them.

Note that mushroom allergy is different from mushroom intolerance. Mushroom allergy triggers your immune system, while mushroom intolerance does not. In mushroom allergy, mushroom antigens can trigger your immune system even if you're yet to eat mushrooms.

Symptoms of Allergic Reaction to Mushroom

You may have gastrointestinal reactions when you have mushroom allergies. The intestine lining becomes inflamed and swollen from the histamine triggered by your body. Other symptoms of mushroom allergies include:

- Nausea

- Light-headedness

- Diarrhea

- Headaches

- Hives

- Shortness of breath

- Cramping

- Wheezing

- Abdominal pain and bloating

Mushroom allergies is a severe medical problem. You might have to see a doctor when you experience these symptoms after eating mushrooms.

Mushroom Intolerance Remedy

Unfortunately, there is no medication that you can use to prevent mushroom intolerance. However, you can stay away from mushroom intake to avoid the discomforting feeling that comes from mushroom intolerance.

Since mushroom intolerance is more about your difficulty with digesting mushrooms and not about your immune system, that would be the best possible remedy.

Now, you know all that you need to know about foraging for mushrooms. You can start looking for edible mushrooms that you can add to your diet for their medicinal and nutritional value. You will learn how to harvest and store mushrooms in the next chapter.

Chapter 4

Harvesting and Storage Tips for Mushrooms

Harvesting your mushroom is a rewarding experience. But it can also be challenging because the process is time-consuming.

The storing process can be even more challenging as it requires careful practice. Learning to do it properly can take a while, but as you practice, you get to know more about the process.

The process begins with harvesting only bright and unblemished mushrooms. It would be best if you chose only mushrooms that look and smell fresh.

Avoid mushrooms that have bad spots, are dry, darkened, shriveled, moldy, have bad spots, and give unpleasant odor. You can't store such mushrooms for long.

When to Harvest Mushrooms

Mushrooms are not like other plants that have an expected growth period. The general rule is to wait patiently to see the mushroom grow out of the compost. The period it takes to grow depends on the type of compost you choose to use, as discussed in the previous chapter.

It also depends, to some extent, on the type of mushroom you choose to grow. However, in about three to four weeks on average, the mushroom should appear. Wait to harvest them when the caps open, that is when the cap turn from convex to concave.

The size of the mushrooms is not an indicator of when to harvest them. Bigger is not always better. You can, however, decide to wait till they become big enough if you prefer it that way.

How to Harvest Mushrooms: Cutting or Picking

There is no big deal about harvesting mushrooms; neither is the process a mystery.

However, there is the debate revolving around which method is best; to pick or to cut the mushroom. The debate as to which technique is best won't end anytime soon, though, as each method has its proponents.

Those who are in support of cutting the mushrooms argue that picking can destroy the surrounding mycelium that is yet to develop or are still developing. They also claim the method resulted in higher yield over time.

Those in support of picking claim that cutting can leave stumps from which diseases can develop and end up contaminating the growing medium.

If you have considered the argument from both sides, which technique should you then choose? The answer is simple because, realistically, there is no difference between the two methods.

They both have their drawbacks, which, if handled properly, would not matter eventually. Therefore, your goal as a mushroom forager is to handle whichever technique you choose to use correctly.

How to Pick or Cut Mushrooms

If you choose to cut mushrooms, only cut with a sharp knife placed at the stem on the mushroom. Also, cut in a way that the stem does not protrude out of the growing system and remember to remove any remaining substrate material.

If you choose to pick the mushroom, place your fingers on the stem and gently pull it out of the substrate. Ensure you carefully separate them from the substrate so that your mushrooms will remain beautiful from the bottom of the stem to the top of the cap.

The goal is to pick the mushrooms in a considerate manner. The key is to be gentle!

For both methods, remember that the mycelium needs to remain active and alive for continuous growth and harvesting.

How to Store Mushrooms

Mushrooms do not last for long before they deteriorate. If you store correctly, they can be useful for up to a week after harvesting them.

If you want to store them for that long, place unwashed mushrooms in a brown paper bag, fold the bag from the top, then place the bag in a cool and dry place.

However, when you need them to stay longer than a week, or you want to sell them off for profit, you have to employ some mushroom preservation methods.

There are two primary mushroom preservation methods you can use, namely; refrigerating or freezing, and drying.

Refrigerating or Freezing

Store them in temperatures between 2 to 4 Celsius to maximize their shelf life. Note that fresh mushrooms do not freeze well, and it won't preserve them from decomposition.

But, if you only need to store fresh mushrooms for a while, wrap them in paper bags and keep in the freezer.

Otherwise, mushrooms should be cooked before you freeze them. That's because cooking kills the enzymes that hasten mushrooms' deterioration process. Therefore, this step is essential, and there are two ways to do it.

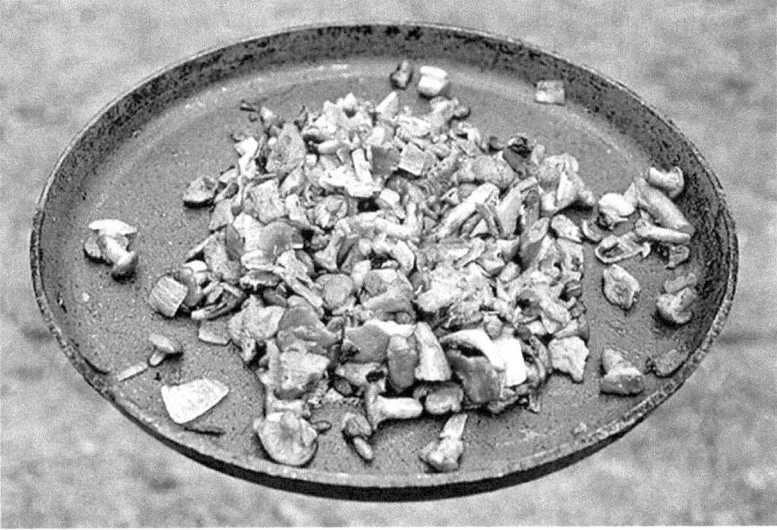

1. Sautéed

When food is sautéed, it means to cook the food in an amount of fat, usually oil, using an open pan.

- Wash the mushrooms in cold water and slice. (don't soak)

- Sauté using butter or oil for about 5 minutes, depending on the number of mushrooms.

- Flash-freeze the mushrooms on a cookie sheet.

- When they are frozen to an extent, transfer them into a container safe for the freezer and keep there.

2. Steamed

Freezing changes the color and texture of the mushrooms, making the mushrooms both dark and soft. Therefore, to reduce the change in color, follow these steps.

- Add lemon juice or citric acid to water in the measurement of one teaspoon to one pint of water.

- Soak the mushrooms in the mixture for about 5 minutes.

- Then, steam for about 5 minutes, depending on the number of mushrooms.

- Flash-freeze on a cookie sheet

- Store in freezer-safe bag or containers.

Drying Mushrooms

Drying your mushrooms is an easy way to preserve them for a long time.

There are several methods you can use to dry your mushrooms. Some of the methods include using a food dehydrator, kitchen oven, the box fan, sun drying, etc.

Whichever method you choose to use, the general process of drying includes the following steps;

- Cut the mushrooms into small sizes. It makes them dry faster.

- Avoid exposing them to too much heat because heat can destroy some of the beneficial components of the mushrooms.

- Check on them regularly to avoid over-drying. The aim is to remove all water contents from the mushrooms. Therefore, they must be crack dry such that they break apart or snap easily.

- Store in an airtight container after drying and leave in a cool, dark place.

- If you're allergic to mushrooms, be careful when you dry them. The heat and air movement can cause spores to move around while drying.

These are the necessary steps for drying your mushrooms. Tweak them to fit the drying method you're using.

Note that too much moisture on your mushrooms can make the drying process tedious. Therefore, avoid washing the mushrooms before you dry them.

Now, you know all that you need to about foraging for mushrooms and harvesting and storing them, you might wonder if there are other plants that you can eat in your region. The next chapter will educate you on wild plants, how to find and recognize them, and harvest and store them.

Chapter 5

Wild Plants

Wild plants are plants that grow on their own. People often consider them as unwanted interference with other plants. Most times, smaller ones are considered as weed and removed from the midst of plants.

The term "wild" is used to describe these plants because they often grow where they are not wanted. They grow spontaneously without human actions.

However, there are edible and medicinal wild plants. Some are aromatic and perfumery.

The benefits of wild plants are numerous and diverse. These plants are a great source of income for farmers. Foragers also take advantage of the gift of nature to gather wild plants. Some edible wild plants can be eaten raw. Some require cooking or drying.

Not all wild plants are edible, though. Some are poisonous and should be avoided.

Wild plants grow in diverse places. A large quantity of them is found in fields, coastal areas, etc. You can learn more about where you can see wild plants.

Where Can Wild Plants Be Found?

There is no restricted growing area for wild plants. They grow anywhere without being planted. These plants do not depend on human nurturing to grow and be productive.

The reality is that gardeners cannot completely get rid of them from their flowerbeds. Even when they do, these plants grow back, or new ones take their place. So, the fight against weed is a continuous one.

Weeds also grow in farms amongst other plants. Because they are unwanted, there are stages in crop farming where the farmers weed them off.

Wild plants are more in abundance in open spaces and wild places like fields, waste places, wetlands, mountains, and hills. They are also found in uninhabited lands and coastal areas.

In these areas, they grow without being cut. These plants also present a pleasant view in these areas because they grow to full size. You might wonder whether wild plants are useful for more than a great view.

Well, hikers and mountaineers forage wild plants. Some people forage as a hobby. However, in some places, it is a survival strategy. Wild plants can be incredibly useful if you know the right use.

Uses of Wild Plants

Since wild plants grow almost on their own, one would think they are not as useful as other plants. However, this assumption is not the case. Wild plants are beneficial all over the world. In rural settings, they play critical economic roles.

• *Economic Gains*

Wild plants contribute to the economic life of any society. This fact is mostly the case in developing countries. Wherever there are agricultural practices, wild plants are essential.

Local communities where agricultural systems flourish mostly depend on wild plants. It is a source of healthy food supply. Tourists, hikers, or mountaineers who forage in these areas gather plenty of foods.

Wild plants are a source of a variety of foods. The roots, stems, leaves, fruits, seeds, tubers, etc. of different plants are edible.

In some places, like Turkey, people eat most wild plants raw. They eat the stalk of Rumex alpinus and Rumex chalepensis raw. However, some plants are either boiled or dried before eating.

Some wild plants go into the making of food additives and processing agents. Bee plants help in producing honey. Wild plants are also used for making wine and beverages.

Some people cook with fuel woods. They cut them from the forest and chop them into usable bits. Some people prefer buying from people who cut them. Farmers usually benefit financially from these plants. Consumers of these products provide a ready market for producers and sellers.

• *Socio-Economic Value*

Wild plants also have socio-economic value. They can be processed and used for dyes, fibers, and shelter. Resins, tannins, latex, oils, wax, etc. are also produced using parts of wild plants.

Cosmetics and perfumes also have parts of plants as their constituting items. Examples of such plants are Achillea spp, Rosemarinus Officinalis, etc.

Wild plants are also used in making medicines for human and animal consumption. These medicines are used in the prevention and treatment of diseases and illnesses.

The importance of medicinal plants cannot be overemphasized. In most communities, these plants are grown close to the home. Some medicinal plants include aloe inermis, Aloe perryi, Salvia fruticosa, etc.

Medicinal plants have been used traditionally from time immemorial. Presently, medicinal plants still play significant roles in the production of drugs. Recent research even unearths the need for these plants.

Most countries, especially developing countries, base their health care on traditional medicines. The World Health Organization (WHO) pens the figures at 80 percent.

Other items produced with wild plants are fuelwood, charcoal, and fertilizer.

The usefulness of wild plants is considered a core of some traditional knowledge. The use of some wild plants is indigenous to some communities. Most times, the culture is preserved and handed down.

Wild plants are essential to nature generally. Some birds and insects depend on them for survival. Some of these insects may go into extinction if these wild plants are not there for them to feed on.

The presence of these wild plants attracts insects. It is a form of natural pest control for farmers. The plants around these wild plants will be free from these insects. Instead, the insect will feed on the wild plants.

Farmers should allow wild plants close to their crops, considering this advantage. The weeds amongst the plants can be taken out, though.

• Beautiful View of Nature
Another fabulous advantage of wild plants is the view they present. Nature has a way of impacting human minds. A pleasant view of the natural environment is beneficial to human well-being.

These advantages of wild plants notwithstanding, some people cut them off. Some farmers and gardens waste no time in cutting them off. If wild plants are preserved, everyone will benefit from it.

Environmental Value of Wild Plants

Wild plants play a unique role in improving the natural environment. Aside from beautification, they help to improve the soil. They also serve as windbreaks. It makes them highly valued in high wind areas.

Wild plants can also help to control erosion. They are also used as ornamentals.

Most people do not fully harness the benefits of wild plants because they see them as disadvantageous. The larger population is not well informed on the merits of having wild plants around.

You should not be a part of this crowd anymore as you have learned the uses of these wild plants. You can start foraging for these plants with the guide that we have provided in the next chapter for locating and identify these plants.

Chapter 6

50 Edible Wide Plants in North America

There are many edible plants that you can forage in North America. However, most of these plants are considered weeds. If you look carefully around you, you'll find several of these edible plants sprouting somewhere close to you.

The next time you're out foraging, don't overlook these nutrient-dense plants. This list will help you to identify what's edible and how to differentiate them from their poisonous varieties.

Chickweed

This plant is an annual herb and often grows on lawns during spring. It doesn't like heat, so you'll find it in shaded areas. It grows on moist grounds.

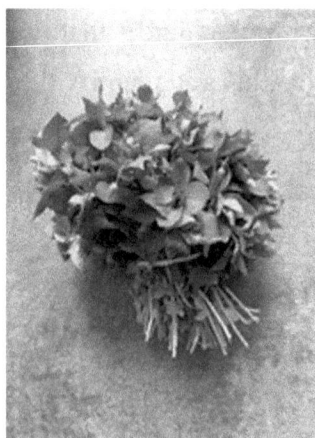

These plants have a distinctive characteristic; the leaves fold up when it about to rain.

Identification

It has five small white-colored, incised flower petals that look like there are ten instead. The slender stem is only hairy on one side and will show up on a different side, after each leave pair.

It has oval-shaped leaves with pointed tips. Unlike other plants, it doesn't have a milky sap.

When opened up, its stem has an elastic pith that won't crease when the outer stem is bent.

The leaves grow in opposite pairs, and the pairs change direction at each node. The older plants often have and can grow up to 12 inches (30 cm) tall.

Edible Parts

Chickweed's flowers, stem, seeds, and leaves are edible.

Safe Consumable Quantity

Eat only a little. Too much of it can upset your stomach.

Best Consumable State

You can eat chickweeds raw or cooked, as a part of stew or soup.

Nutritional Value

Chickweeds are rich in minerals and vitamins. It's a rich source of vitamin C, potassium, calcium, selenium, magnesium, beta-carotene, etc.

Location

It can be found in open fields and lawns.

Fireweed

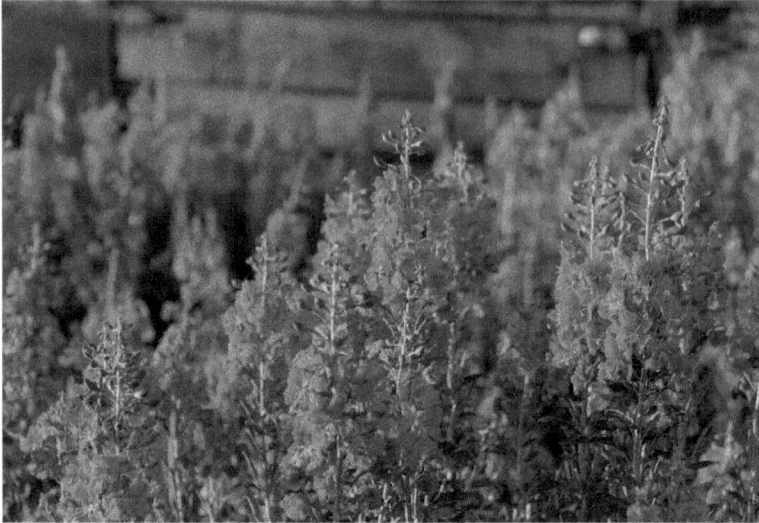

This pretty looking plant could be mistaken for just another flower that brightens the field where it grows. However, it's an edible plant to snack on when you need food in the wild.

In Britain, the plant is called the Rosebay Willow Herb or the Great Willow Herb.

Identification

It has a plain, smooth reddish stem with its lance-shaped leaves alternating each other in a scattered pattern. The fireweed flower is large and pinkish, with four petals and stigmas. The plants grow very tall, as dwarf species can be as high as 12 to 14 inches (20-60cm) tall.

It has a circular patterned vein structure. This feature makes it unique and easy to differentiate from other toxic lily plants in early spring when they tend to look alike.

Edible Parts

You can eat the flower, leaves, and stem in early spring. They tend to taste bitter and are tougher in summer.

The pith of older plants can be eaten raw, so you can also split the stem open to extract it.

You can also eat the roots, after roasting and scraping off its outer layer, but it has a bitter taste.

Safe Consumable Quantity

You can eat as much as you like.

Best Consumable State

You can eat fireweed shoots raw or cooked when its leaves are ready to eat. You can pickle or sauté the shoots.

Nutritional Value

It's rich in Vitamin A and C.

Location

You'll find fireweeds on stream banks, open woods, hillside, seashores in the artic, open fields, and pastures, and alpine slopes.

Wood Sorrels

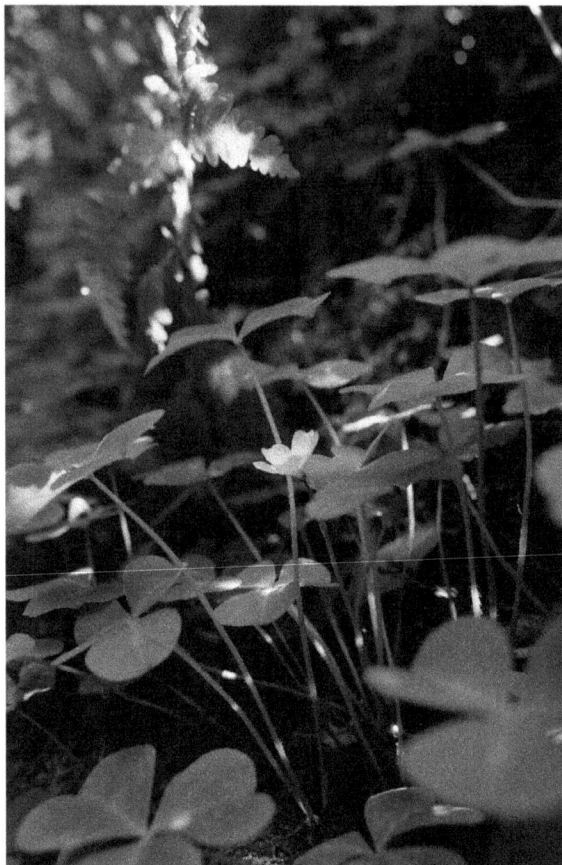

These plants come in different varieties and often bloom through spring and fall. It has a mild lemony taste that will quench your thirst when you're out in the wild.

Identification

The plant has a compound leave structure with three heart-shaped leaflets folded along the mid-vein. They can come in shades of purple or burgundy, although most are green colored. These leaves fold up at night and open up in the morning and may fold up under harsh sunlight too.

Its flowers with five petals can be white or yellowish. At the same time, some other varieties may have violet or pinkish colored petals.

Its seedpods point outward at about 90 degrees from the stalk it grows on. Stalks also grow at about the same angle from the main stem.

Edible Parts

You can eat all parts of this plant. Its leaves, seeds pods resembling tiny okra fruits, flowers, and roots are edible.

Safe Consumable Quantity

Eat-in moderation, as the high oxalic content can be toxic.

Best Consumable State

You can eat wood sorrel raw or add it as a seasoning in your food. It could also be used as a coffee flavor, or as part of your salad.

Nutritional Value

The Wood Sorrel is rich in vitamin C. Some species are edible tuber plants, rich in fiber, amino acids, and proteins.

Location

You'll find wood sorrels in the woods and on forest floors.

Mustard Greens

If you find this invasive weed anywhere close to you, then it's time to fetch them to serve some purpose for your belly. You'll find it garlic-like taste an excellent addition in your meals.

Identification

The leaves of these plants are kidney-shaped or heart-shaped depending on how close the leaves carve in at the midvein. Its edges come off in a sharp, irregular pattern, although it might appear scalloped in younger leaves. The leaves of this plant may or may not be hairy.

The flower has five white petals, six stamens, and four green sepals. You'll often find four of the stamens tall, and the other two are short. The flowers usually bloom between May and June.

Edible Parts

The seeds, roots, stem, flowers, and leaves of the mustard green are edible.

Safe Consumable Quantity

Eat the leaves in moderation, or soak in water before eating because of its cyanide content.

Best Consumable State

It's best to eat garlic mustard leaves in cool weather as they become bitter when the weather is hot. But, the leaves are edible regardless of the season of the year.

You can add the flowers to your salads and gather their seeds for eating during fall. The spicy roots can also be collected at the beginning of spring or towards the end of fall. You could also add the stem to your veggies when the plant is yet to flower.

Nutritional Value

Green mustards are rich in Vitamin A, E, C, and Beta-carotene. It also has high fiber content and contains manganese, calcium, iron, and zinc.

Location

Garlic Mustard can be found around swamps, ditches, disturbed forest floors, roadsides, and fence lines. It is common in many parts of the U.S. and Canada.

Wild Black Cherries

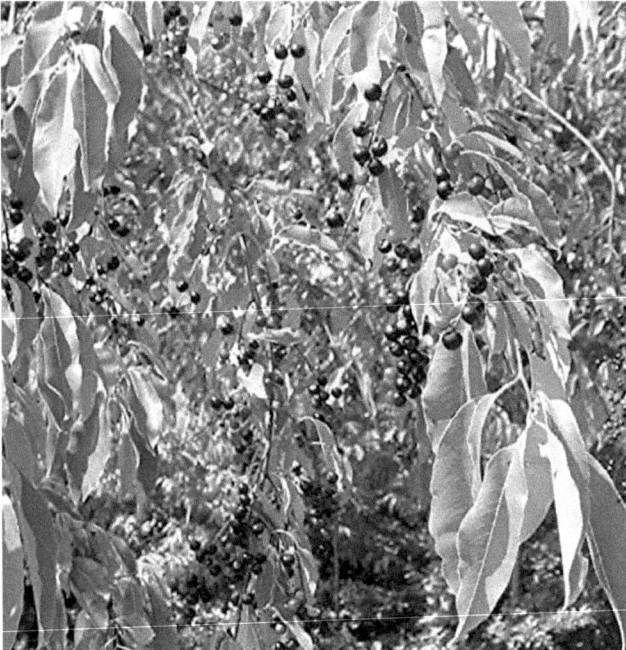

These nice-looking fruits in rich in flavor and provide a tasty snack for those lucky enough to find some. You'll find its reddish or blackish-purple drupe inviting when it fully matures at early fall.

Identification

The leaves of these plants come off in an ovate pattern, lining alternatively along the branches of the trees. It's usually about 6 inches long.

The tree has a smooth, light brown bark, which could become darker and rougher with age. The branches are long and slender and may grow long enough to touch the ground.

You'll find the cluster of flowers at the end of the plant's branches. On a closer look, the white flowers have five petals, with five sepals and several stamens. They bud on a raceme of about 4-6 inches long.

The fruits show up at the end of the raceme after the flower bloom is over, appearing green, turning to dark red, and eventually purplish-black at full maturity.

Edible Parts

The fruits are edible, although it may taste bitter.

Safe Consumable Quantity

It's safe to consume this fruit only in moderation because of its seed's cyanide content.

Best Consumable State

It can be eaten raw or pressed out for its juice.

Nutritional Value

Wild black cherries can be a good source of vitamin C and provide useful antioxidants to the body.

Location

You'll mostly find various species in many parts of Canada and the USA. You could stumble on one in a park, field, or open forest.

Alfalfa

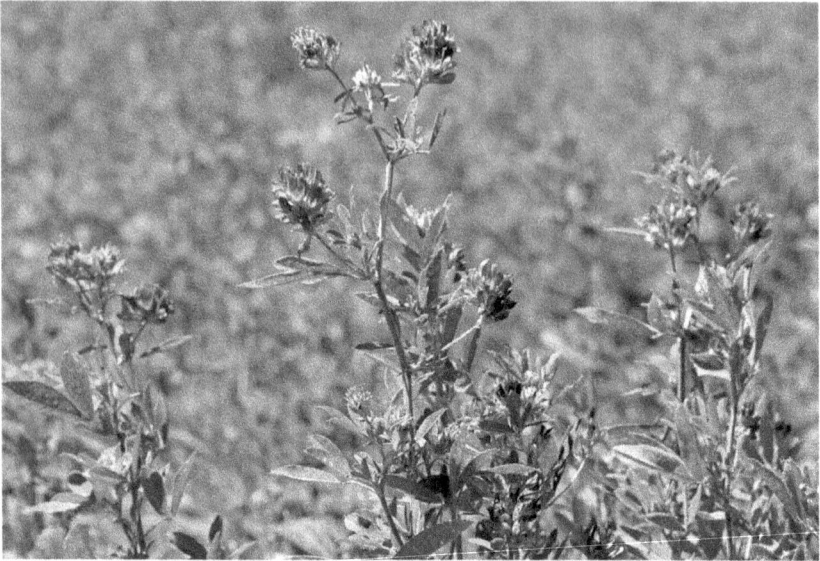

If you find yourself trying to pick out wild herbs for food, Alfalfa is one herb you can find out there. It is highly rated for its medicinal advantages and planted by some people. You can be lucky to find it growing somewhere around you by itself.

Identification

You'll find this plant growing on a moist to wet ground but not in a shed. It can grow up to 1m in height, and you'll find it flowering between June to July, with seeds maturing through July to September.

The Alfalfa's leaves are divided into three narrow leaflets with serrated edges. The middle leaflet protrudes outward than the others.

The purple flowers grow in clusters on a raceme and can contain between 10 to 30 flowers per cluster.

Its seed pods grow spiral and may contain up to 6 seeds in a pod.

Edible Parts

You can eat the leaves, seeds, and shoots of the Alfafa.

Safe Consumable Quantity

It's best to eat only a little of this plant, even if you find it in abundance around you. It may pose potential risks to the red blood cells.

Best Consumable State

The leaves are edible, either eaten raw or cooked. You might want to boil it considerably to reduce its saponin content. The seeds could be used in the sprouted form in salads.

Nutritional Value

The plant is rich in protein, vitamins A, B, C, and K (the leaves)

Location

It is commonly found in meadows, woodlands, disturbed fields, and riversides.

Dandelions

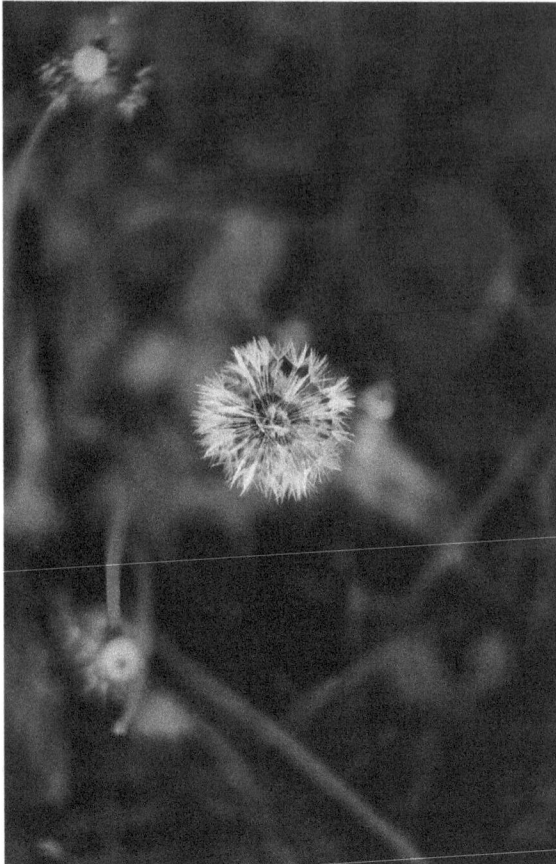

The beautiful flowers of this plant make it easy to spot amidst other weeds.

Identification

Dandelions grow as close as possible to the ground. The leaves shoot out at about 90 degrees from the stem and not upwards, like in some resembling species.

The leaves have sharp tooth-like edges that are smooth. They don't have hair on their surface, and the stems may produce milky sap. The stems are often whitish but may possess a purplish color.

The flowers are bright yellow, as is the case in any sunflower specie. Although, it might be challenging to identify dandelions with their flowers because many other varieties share the same flower structure.

Edible Parts

The leaves and roots are edible.

Safe Consumable Quantity

Eat dandelions in moderation. You should also avoid it as a pregnant or nursing mother.

Best Consumable State

It is best eaten raw or slightly cooked to preserve its nutrient base. It could also be dried and powdered to flavor food.

Nutritional Value

It's rich in Vitamin K, beta-carotene, calcium, omega-fatty acids, amongst other beneficial minerals.

Location

It is common to grassy areas and disturbed zones.

Curly Dock

Finding a tender curly dock plant while foraging, can make all the efforts worth it. You'll find a rich green vegetable, tasting like spinach, when you stumble on the tender one.

Identification

The leaves of this plant are long, narrow, and curly, as the name implies. They grow close to the ground and high up on the stem. However, the leaves at the bases are longer and broader than those on the stem.

You may find a whitish sheath around the nodes, which will eventually turn brown with age.

The flowers, often purplish, can number up to 25 in a cluster. They are usually small and nearly insignificant.

The seeds grow on the stalk enclosed in a leaf-like capsule. They are often three-sided, with a side pointing outwards sharply. The seeds' case may become brown with age, but it often remains on the stalk through winter.

Edible Parts

The curly dock leaves, stem, seeds, and roots are edible.

You can harvest the stem before it flowers for a rich taste. It is best to collect the freshly unfurled leaves for better taste. The seeds can also be processed, and the roots harvested.

Safe Consumable Quantity

It's best to eat curly docks in moderation to avoid ingesting too much oxalic acid.

Best Consumable State

You can eat it raw or cooked depending on the season of harvest or the part of the plant you're eating.

Nutritional Value

It's rich in vitamins B, A, and C, and iron.

Location

You'll find this plant around roadsides, construction sites, and disturbed fields.

Chicory

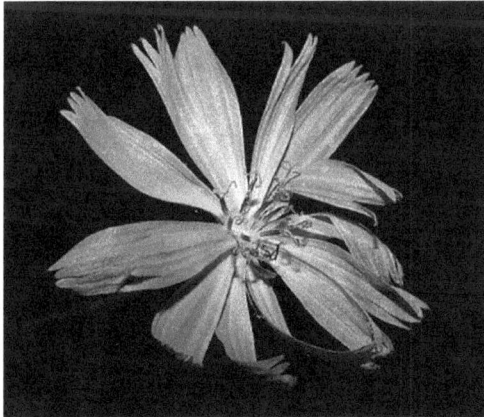

This plant is a common weed that you must have come across in many places, especially on roadsides. It's beautiful edible flowers can be inviting when in full bloom.

Identification

The leaves often grow pointed from the harsh, hairy stem. They grow in alternate patterns and are lance-shaped. The leaves are often broader towards the base, and all have lobed edges.

You'll find the flowers have a sky blue, pink, or white color, and only open up when it's sunny. They are parallel-shaped and overlap over each other.

The stem has a milky sap, and the leaves grow thinner upward. The plant has a tap root system.

Edible Parts

You can eat all parts of this plant. The leaves, stem, flowers, and roots are edible.

Safe Consumable Quantity

Any quantity of Chicory roots and leaves added to a meal is safe. If you're eating it raw, then you might have to deal with its bitter taste in the amounts you eat them. It's not considered safe for pregnant women, though.

Best Consumable State

You can eat this plant raw, but you can boil it to reduce its bitter taste.

Nutritional Value

It contains B-vitamins and is highly rich in fiber.

Location

It is a common weed in North America. It can be found in old fields, roadsides, and weedy areas.

Creeping Charlie

You can be lucky to find this nutritious green while you're out hiking in the woods.

Identification

The leaves grow on long stalks, have a round or kidney-shaped, and scalloped edges. They grow in pairs on the stems and tend to be greener than the plant towards the upper parts of the stem. The leaves have a sparse hairy surface.

The plant stem is square, and the root is fibrous. The stems carrying the flower stand more erect and have smaller leaves on them.

The plant generally forms a mat on the floor and can establish another root, if a node on the stem, touches the floor. The plant grows rapidly when it finishes flowering.

The flowers often have a blue to purplish color and have their two-lipped petals in a tube-like form. You'll find the flowers clustered in threes.

Edible Parts

The young leaves of this plant are edible and will add a minty taste to your meals.

Safe Consumable Quantity

As long as you eat Creeping Charlie in moderation, you are at no risk.

Best Consumable State

You can eat it raw or cooked.

Nutritional Value

Creeping Charlie is rich in vitamin C.

Location

You'll find Creeping Charlie in moist areas, shady areas, lawns, and edges of woodland.

Harebell

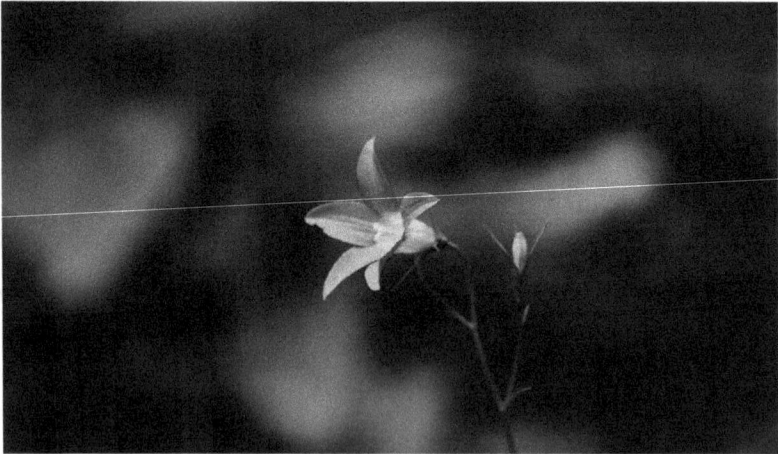

It is commonly called bluebells or lady's thimble. It looks far from edible but can be a good source of food. If you find this plant while foraging, don't hesitate to pick some for food.

Identification

The leaves of this plant are often kidney-shaped and can be up to 7cm longs at maturity. The leaves at the base of the plant are often round. Those at the top of the stem are usually thinner and grass-like.

The sap of the plant is milky and flows when the leaves or stem is broken. The stem is narrow and may even hang downwards due to its light-weight.

Its flowers are bell-shaped, probably the reason why it's called bluebells. The purple flowers bloom on the thicker stalk with narrow leaves. They have five spoon-shaped lobes on its outer edges.

You'll find the flower blooms from June through September.

Edible Parts

The leaves of this plant are edible.

Best Consumable State

You can eat the leaves raw as a part of your salads or cooked with your meals.

Nutritional Value

This plant is famous for its rich vitamin C content.

Location

Harebells are common to wooded areas, meadows, beaches, shaded and open areas. They are common in most parts of the USA and Canada.

Broadleaf Plantain

This plant is another exotic edible weed. On the surface, it may appear scary looking, but you have free food if you ever find it.

Identification

It is known by its large leaves, oval in shape, and thick stems. The stems grow out from a base. The flowers are greenish, long, with erect spikes that grow from the leaves at the bottom.

The flowers have four petals, a pistil, and two stamens. The seeds form below the flowers.

Edible Parts

Broadleaf plantain leaves and seeds are edible and have a lot of medicinal uses.

Safe Consumable Quantity

The seeds may cause bloating, so don't overeat it.

Best Consumable State

The leaves can be cooked, or it can be eaten raw. It has a bitter taste, and it can be a bit of work harvesting the seeds.

Nutritional Value

These plants contain tannins, flavonoids, and glycosides, which are all anti-inflammatory compounds that can help to reduces inflammation.

Location

You can find broadleaf plantain on playgrounds, walkways, and open fields.

Pineapple Weed

It is an annual plant that is often mistaken for chamomile. It has a pineapple-like odor when crushed.

Identification

It is a low-growing plant with finely divided foliage that emits a pineapple smell when crushed. Pineapple weed has a cone-shaped flower head that is greenish-yellow in color.

The leaves are finely divided into narrow, feathery segments. They can grow up to 2 to 4cm and are hairless.

The entire plant grows to about 30cm tall.

Edible Parts

The flower and leaves are edible.

Safe Consumable Quantity

The tea from pineapple weed can be taken every night.

Best Consumable State

The flowers can be dried out and crushed to be used as flour. The leaves are useful as tea.

Nutritional Value

This weed can cure fever, stomach upset, and insomnia. It also contains analgesic properties and is highly recommended for breastfeeding mothers.

Location

This plant grows in between sidewalk cracks and almost all waste areas and it can even survive in abused soil such as driveways, dirt roads, and sandy soil. It's common to North America.

Mallow

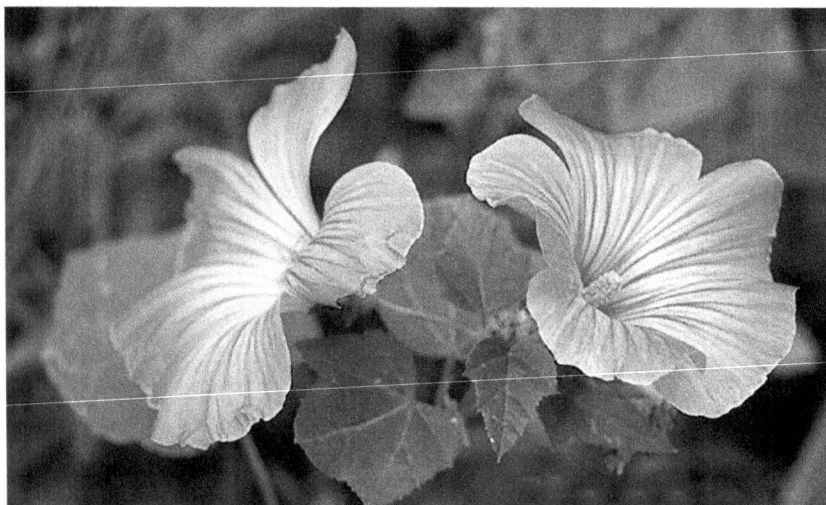

If you know the hibiscus flower or hollyhock, then you can recognize a Mallow plant. The only difference is its broad leaves.

Identification

The leaves are round and distinct. The flowers and seed pods are small and round, often blurred by the leaves. Mallow has a funnel-shaped flower with five petals and a unique column of stamens surrounding the pistil.

The fruits are round and have cheese-like wedges. The stems are flexible and come from a central point, lounging on the ground.

The stem originates from a deep taproot and is low spreading with branches that can be up to 60cm long.

The flowers are borne either singly or in clusters from the axils.

Edible Parts

The leaves, stems, flowers, seeds, and roots are edible.

Safe Consumable Quantity

It's best to consume it in a reasonable quantity.

Best Consumable State

You can eat it raw or cooked like vegetables.

Nutritional Value

Mallow is rich in calcium, magnesium, and iron

Location

You'll find this plant in most parts of North America. This plant grows in lawns, gardens, roadsides, or waste areas.

Coneflower

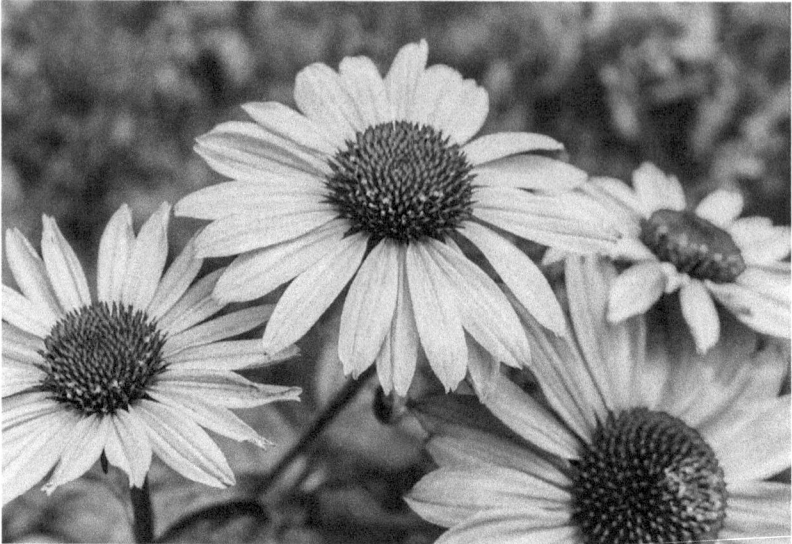

This fast-growing plant sows its seeds and is easy to grow. You can find them in bright, purple, or subdued colors to suit your garden.

Identification

Coneflowers are easy to identify. The flower is rounded and stand upright. It has larger lower leaves than the upper leaves.

The stem is stiff and has thin, vertical, purple lines on it. The stems branch into lateral limbs or remain straight and unbranched.

The leaves emerge alternately and singly from the stem and are lance-shaped. They have cone-like centers that contain seeds that attract butterflies.

Coneflowers are drought tolerant and trouble-free.

Edible Parts

All parts of the coneflower are edible, but the leaves and flower buds are used for herbal tea.

Safe Consumable Quantity

You can take as much as you want.

Best Consumable State

The flower and leaves are dried to make herbal tea.

Nutritional Value

It has positive effects on the immune system, lowers blood sugar level, reduces anxiety, and cures cold and skin cancer.

Location

It's common in most parts of North America.

Elderberry

This dark purple berry comes from the European elder tree. It is often confused with American Elder, Dwarf Elder, or Elderflower, but they're not the same.

Identification

Look for clusters of small white flowers, drooping purple fruit, and hard, woody bark. Elderberry commonly grows in a bushy, shrub-like pattern. Mature elderberry plants can be as tall as 9 to 12 feet or 2.7 to 3.7m.

Elderberry love to grow in moist habitats.

Edible Parts

The fruits, flowers, and the petals of these plants are edible.

Safe Consumable Quantity

The fruits can be eaten as much as you want. But when made into tea, it should not be taken more than three times a day.

Best Consumable State

The fruits and petals are eaten raw. The flower can be dipped in batter and fried.

Nutritional Value

It is high in Vitamin C and dietary fiber.

Location

You can find elderberries on the stream banks, marshes, or moist forests.

Meadowsweet

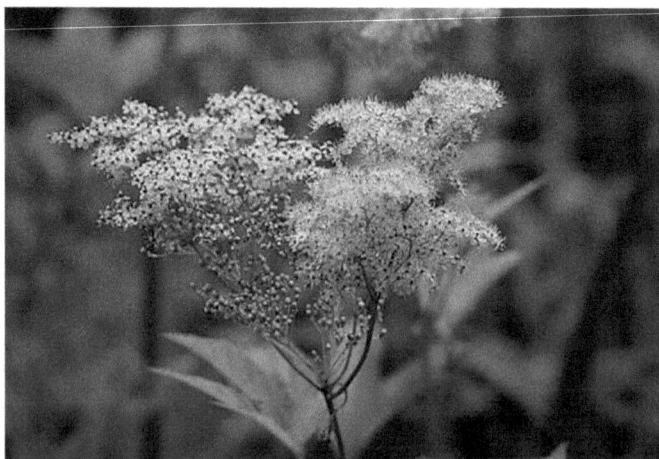

This plant is the prettiest and the most fragrant of all hedgerow plants. It has creamy yellow flowers and spreads honey, vanilla, and almond scents in the neighborhood.

Identification

The tree grows as high as a meter or two meters. The dark green leaves have up to 3 to 5 pairs of toothed leaflets with smaller leaves around them. The upper surface is smooth, and the undersides are somewhat hairy.

The flower has a pleasant scent when they open for the first time. The smell becomes stronger when the flowers fade.

The stems and leaves also have a fragrance, but it is not as sharp as that of the flowers.

Edible Parts

Its leaves, blossoms, buds, and seeds are edible.

Safe Consumable Quantity

It is safe in low quantities, as a high dose can act as an anticoagulant and prevent blood clotting.

Best Consumable State

The leaves can be eaten raw or cooked as a green.

Nutritional Value

It's rich in carbohydrates, sugars, and Vitamin C.

Location

It's common to most parts of North America.

Pepper Grass

This plant of the mustard family has a spicy flavor. It is an excellent addition to salads, soups, pasta, and other dishes.

Identification

This plant has a raceme that comes from the plant's highly branched stem. Flowers grow at the top of the racemes.

This plant has tiny white flowers with four petals, two to four stamens, and can be 1 to 3mm long. It has four cupped, greenish-white sepals about 1mm long.

The leaves are lance-shaped and hairy. The leaves are basal at the base of the plant and can grow up to 2 to 15cm long with a large terminal lobe and various lateral lobes.

Edible Parts

The entire plant is edible.

Safe Consumable Quantity

Eat as you deem fit.

Best Consumable State

Mix the leaves with salad or grind the roots to make tea.

Nutritional Value

It contains protein, iron, vitamin A, and C.

Location

The plants are common to North America. The plant can be found along roadsides, disturbed sites, pastures, and waste areas.

Field Pennycress

Field pennycress is also known as Stinkweed, Frenchweed, or Fanweed. It may occur as either a winter or summer annual plant.

Identification

The seeds are oval-shaped & dark brown. They are rounded at one point and taperer to a point at the other end.

The stems are ribbed and may be winged along the ribs. The alternate leaves are up to 4 inches long and 1 inch across. The leaf margins appear wavy and sometimes can have blunt teeth.

The root system is that of a taproot. The flowers are tiny, about ⅛ inches across when fully open, with four white petals and four green sepals.

Edible Parts

The seeds and leaves are edible.

Safe Consumable Quantity

Large doses can cause a decrease in white blood cells. It is not safe during pregnancy and breastfeeding.

Best Consumable State

The leaves can be eaten raw or boiled.

Nutritional Value

It's rich in protein, fat, carbohydrate, and oil.

Location

Field Pennycress is commonly found in nursery plots, areas along railroads and roadsides, fallow fields, gardens, and cropland.

Purple Deadnettle

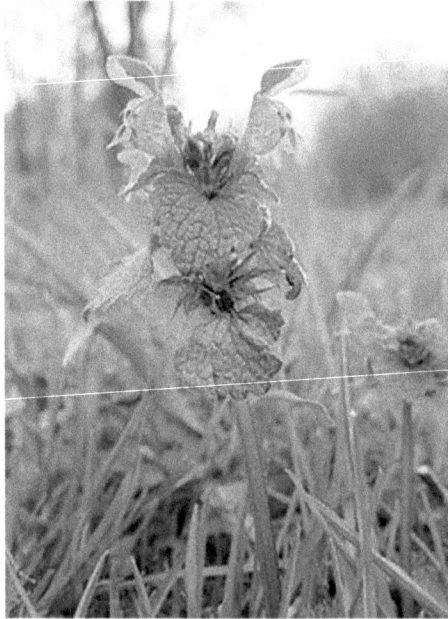

This plant is also known as "devouring purple monster." It was given the name to describe its effect in the winter season as its purple color can turn an entire field into purple in winter.

Identification

It is an annual plant. The hairy nettle doesn't sting, hence the name "dead nettle." You'll commonly find it around wastelands and sidewalks.

The plant has triangular-shaped leaves with the stalk joining the blade of the stem. The flowers are pink in color, with a tube-like shape. The lower and upper ends incline towards one another.

The stems are square in shape, with a mixture of greenish color at the bottom and shades of purple at the top.

Edible Parts

The deadnettle leaves are the only edible part of the plant.

Best Consumable State

The leaves can be used in salad, blended as smoothies, for soups, and also for tea. So, you can choose to consume it raw or cooked.

Best Consumable Quantity

Eat the leaves in moderation.

Nutritional Value

It can be of good medicinal use. It contains anti-inflammatory, anti-fungal, and anti-bacterial properties.

Location

You'll find purple deadnettle in most gardens in North America.

Forget Me Not

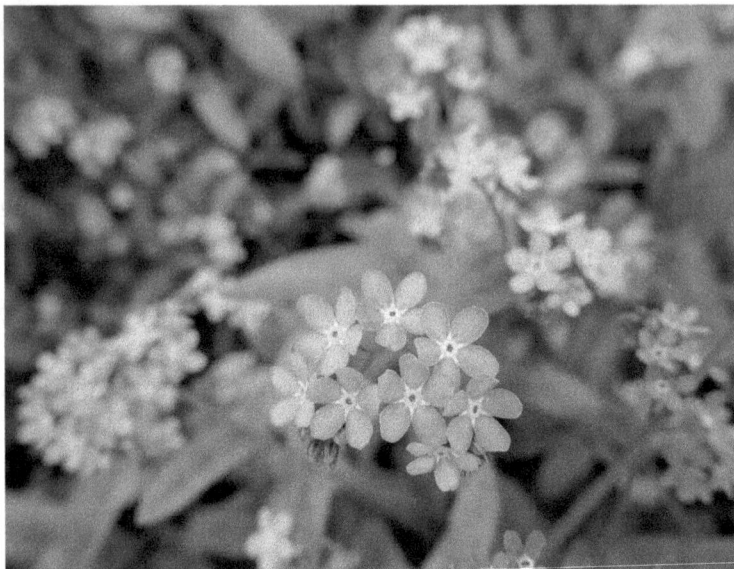

This flower is known to symbolize true love. The flowers are used to decorate gifts with the hope that the recipients will not forget the giver. The flowers give out a lovely fragrance during the evening.

Identification

The flowers have 3 to 5mm greyish-blue petals. The curved flowering stalks open up to display a succession of five-lobed flowers.

The leaves and stems are soft and hairy. The upper leaves have no stalks and alternate along the stem. The plant's branch can grow to a height of 40cm.

The fruits are mericarp egg-shaped and at 1.5 to 2mm long. They are glossy, narrow-winged, and yellowish-brown in color.

The plant is commonly seen on roadside verges, woodland edges, crumbling walls, and hedgerows.

Edible Parts

The flowers of this plant are edible.

Safe Consumable Quantity

The flowers are non-toxic and can be eaten as often as you want.

Best Consumable State

The flowers can be eaten raw as a snack or tossed in a salad or used to decorate desserts and garnish your meals.

Nutritional Value

The whole plant is used as medicine and can cure nosebleeds and lung problems.

Location

The plant is common in North America, and some species are native to California.

Mullein

This plant is characterized by its soft leaves and yellow flowers at the top that gives it a unique appearance.

Identification

This soft biennial plant grows tall. It produces leaves in a rosette shape during its first year of growth.

The tall stem looks like a pole and has a dense spike of yellow flowers. It spreads the seeds it produces, but it is not aggressively invasive. Its seeds germinate on open ground.

The flowers grow to 5 to 60cm long, and each flower has five petals, hairy green sepals, stamens, and one pistil. A seed capsule replaces each flower with two cells and numerous tiny seeds.

The large oval-shaped leaves form a basal rosette. It comes in a gray-green color and the leaves grow up to 50cm in length.

Edible Parts

You can eat the leaves and flowers.

Safe Consumable Quantity

You can eat this weed as often as you want.

Best Consumable State

The leaves and flowers can be eaten as a salad and boiled to make tea.

Nutritional Value

Its rich in antioxidants used to cure a common cold and asthma. It's also good for muscle relief.

Location

It's common to the United States and Southern Canada. Mullein is found in open fields, railway embankments, disturbed areas, and waste places.

Bull Thistle

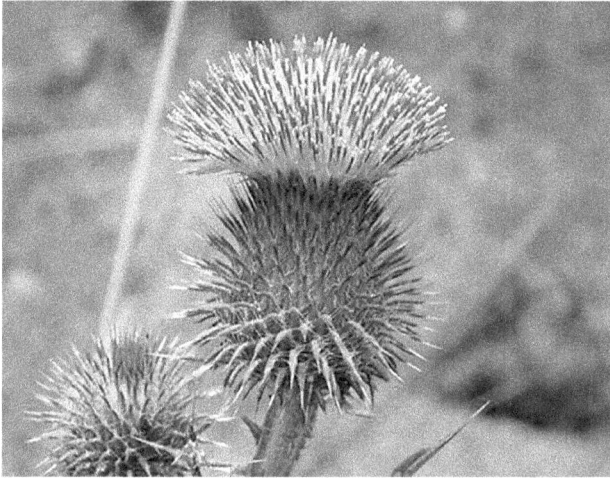

This plant is covered with short, sharp prickles on the top and dark-green leaf blade. It is difficult to touch the surface because of the prickles.

Identification

The flower heads are purple and grow up to 3.5 to 5cm in diameter, and 2.5 to 5cm in length. The flowers have narrow, spine-tipped bracts.

The leaves are alternate and lance-shaped. They have rough, bristle hairs on top and underneath. The leaves measure up to 7.5 to 30cm long.

The stem is firm and thorny. It yields numerous seeds with small feathers and is attached to the base by a ring till they ripen. It tends to grow and survive in disturbed areas and areas with moderate moisture.

Edible Parts

The root, flower stems, leaves, flower buds, and seeds are edible.

Safe Consumable Quantity

Eat as you deem fit. But, avoid its thorny parts.

Best Consumable State

The root can be mixed with other vegetables. The flower stems can be cooked, and the young leaves can be eaten in a salad. The flower buds can be prepared, and the seeds can be roasted.

Nutritional Value

It's rich in inulin and protein. It is also good at curing liver problems and type II diabetes.

Location

Bull thistle is common and can be found in most parts of North America.

Kudzu

This vine is known for its fast and wild growth. It is a highly invasive species that grows up to 30cm per day.

Identification

The leaves form with three leaflets attached to each node. The leaves are connected to the stem on their stalk. The central leaf's petiole is about 19mm long, and the other two have shorter petioles.

The long vines have small, brownish bristles that trail on the ground or climb vertical surfaces. They can cover a whole tree or entire building structures. The thick vines are woody.

The flowers are purple or reddish-purple and are arranged in clusters. The flowers can grow up to 8 inches high.

Edible Parts
The leaves, vine tips, flowers, and roots are edible.

Safe Consumable Quantity
A little portion of it should be eaten the first time to know if you're allergic to it. If not, you can consume as much as you want.

Best Consumable State
The leaves can be eaten raw, chopped, baked, or deep-fried. The root is often made into a tea.

Nutritional Value
It's rich in calories, protein, carbohydrates, fiber, and fat.

Location
It is found in the Southeastern United States.

Pickerelweed
This aquatic plant has its leaves and flowers above water and part of the stem underwater.

Identification

You can find this plant in shallow waters. It has one spike of small flowers and heart-shaped leaves and the flower stem rises above the leaves, with just one leaf growing behind the flowers.

The flowers bloom following each other from the bottom to the top. This flowering method prolongs the flowering period for several days. The flowers grow as high as 6 inches.

The large leaves provide a habitat for fish, birds, reptiles, and swimming mammals.

Its dense root system provides a wave barrier that keeps the shoreline sediment from erosion. The leaves measure up to 10 to 25cm and have long petioles.

Edible Parts

The seeds and the leaves are edible.

Safe Consumable Quantity

The nuts can be eaten as much as you want, but be sure that the water source you harvested the weed from is not polluted.

Best Consumable State

The seeds can be eaten like nuts, and the leaf-stalks cooked as green.

Nutritional Value

It's rich in vitamins and minerals.

Location

This plant can be found in most parts of North America.

Red Clover

The red clover is an edible plant belonging to the legume family. Its history dates back to the Chinese, who used it for medicinal purposes. Native Americans and other notable cultures also believed it to be a potent cure for burns and bronchial problems.

Identification

Red clover has a distinctive appearance because of its reddish flower. Its head is made up of different tubular-shaped flowers. It has green leaves made up of pale green or white chevron at the upper side of the plant. This feature protects the plant from pollinator's insects.

The leaves are oval and are generally broader in the middle of the plant. The base of each compound leaf contains a pair of stipules.

Edible Parts

Red clover gives the best taste among other types of clovers. The flower is the most edible part of the red clover. The leaves can also be added to salad or tea for consumption.

Safe Consumable Quantity

It's best to eat it in moderation, to avoid side effects like nausea, rash, or headache.

Best Consumable State

It is advisable not to overeat the flower because it might cause bloating.

Nutritional Value

It's rich in vitamin C and a good source of minerals like potassium, phosphorus, calcium, and magnesium.

Location

It's common to most parts of North America. They are typically found among pastures, fields and can grow to about 80 centimeters in length.

Partridgeberry

Partridgeberry belongs to the madder family with stems spanning to about 20 centimeters in length. It is characterized by its pair of white tubular flowers with red berries. They are also called twinberry.

Identification

The stems of the plants are generally light green to light brown. They later become brown and smoothens as it grows old. The flowers are radially symmetrical, measuring about 13-16 mm in length.

The flowers are located at either the axils of leaves or tips of the branches. Each of the flower pairs shares the same tubular calyx.

Partridgeberry leaves are oval with smooth surfaces along its margins. It is made up of a shiny upper surface with a dark green color.

Edible Parts

The berries and the leaves of the plant are edible, but the leaves are usually made into a tea. The fruit has a bland taste and can be used in any culinary dish.

Safe Consumable Quantity

It's relatively safe to consume, but should be avoided by pregnant women and breastfeeding mothers.

Best Consumable State

You can use the leaves dried in tea and eat the flesh of the berry.

Nutritional Value

It's rich in protein, fiber, and calories.

Location

They are usually found in rocky upland, sandy savannas, and slopes of wooded ravines. It's particularly common to eastern North America.

Sheep Sorrel

Sheep Sorrel is one of the most common wild edible plants across North America. It is a perennial plant belonging to the Buckwheat family. It grows by spreading out its horizontal roots and bringing out seeds. They have an average height of about 10 to 40 cm.

Identification

It can easily be identified by its arrow-shaped leaves, which usually grow like a rosette. A creeping root system joins the growing leaves underground. The sheep sorrel belongs to a similar specie as the dock seed, and the similarity shows in their seed heads.

They usually grow in patches because of their creeping root. The flowers are unisexual, with the male types having a yellowish color. In contrast, females have a reddish-green color. They are small and have whorls with a branching cluster.

The bottom of the leaves is lobed out, unlike the common sorrel, which has a pointed leaf base. The middle leaves have a lateral lobe on either side and are short-stalked.

Edible Parts

The leaves are edible. Foragers usually use it as thickeners in soups or ground it as flour to make noodles. It tastes like citrus or apple peel and has a lemon or tart flavor.

Safe Consumable Quantity

It's best consumed in moderate amounts. Overeating could be nauseating.

Best Consumable State

The leaves can either be eaten raw or cooked.

Nutritional Value

The plant is rich in vitamin C.

Location

It's common in forest areas of North America.

Shepherds Purse

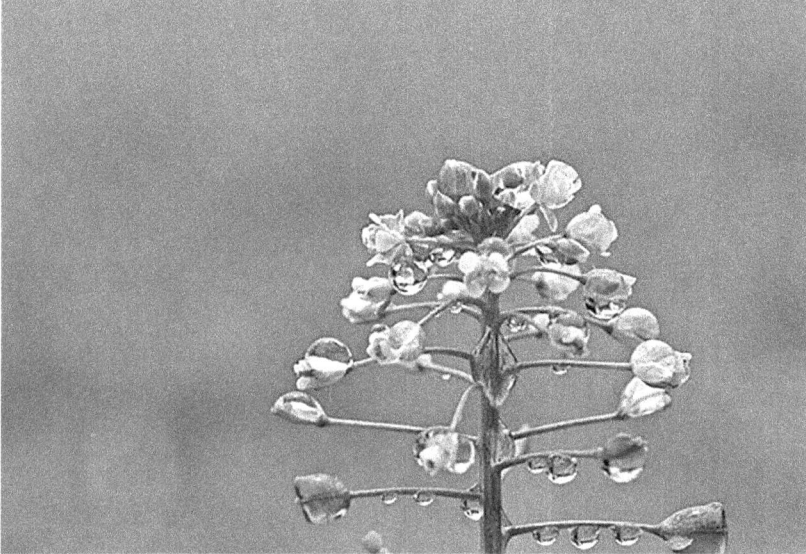

The shepherds' purse usually appears early in the Spring. As the plant begins to grow flowers, the basal leaves will start to wither, leaving just the smaller leaves.

Identification

Their purse-shaped seedpods can quickly identify them. It belongs to the mustard family and can be differentiated from others by its lobed basal leaves. The leaves grow to about 10 cm in length.

The first set of leaves to grow are usually rounded while the later set of leaves are deeply toothed. Shepherds purse often grows to an average height of about 30cm.

Edible Parts

It can be substituted as cabbage or cress in salads. Both the shepherd purse seeds and the flowering shoots are also edible parts of the wild plant. Drying the root can be substituted as ginger for consumption.

Generally, the leaves are available throughout the year, and they can be dried for later use.

Safe Consumable Quantity

Consume moderate quantities, and pregnant women should avoid it.

Best Consumable State

The leaves can either be consumed raw or cooked, depending on your choice.

Nutritional Value

It's rich in iron, vitamin C, and calories.

Location

The plant is common in most parts of North America. They are usually found in grain fields, roadsides, waste areas, and gardens.

Sunflower

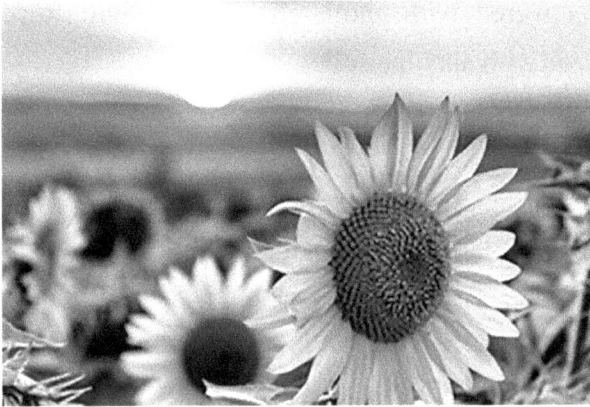

The wild sunflower has a showy ray petal which usually attracts butterflies and birds. You can call them the non-cultivated version of the sunflower.

The sunflower's main source of nutrition comes from photosynthesis production and that is why the sunflower and its leaves turn to follow the sun – they are phototropic.

Identification

They are annual plants with hairy, coarse, and leafy features. They generally grow to a height of about 1.5 meters with a stiff and upright stalk. You will quickly notice them from their yellow florets.

A reddish-brown central disc is located at the top of the flower. About 40 to 80 ray florets surround the flowers.

Their leaves have a scratchy and rough texture, which can measure up to about 30cm in length. Short, stiff hairs are scattered across the upper part of the leaves. They have a light green to reddish petioles which are covered with short, stiff hairs. Sunflowers generally thrive in areas with alkaline soil.

Edible Parts

You can also ground it into powder and mix it with flour for bread. The leaves petioles can be boiled with other vegetables for consumption.

Safe Consumable Quantity

Eat the seeds in your desired quantity.

Best Consumable State

The seeds can either be consumed raw or cooked.

Nutritional Value

They are rich in protein, Vitamin E, and magnesium.

Location

They are usually found in waste areas, fences, roads, and fields.

Spring Beauty

Spring beauty, also known as Claytonia carolianais, develops from a starchy rhizome. Energy from previous seasons is stored in the rhizome to propel its growth early in the Spring.

This wild plant uses the yellow circle and the pink veins on the flowers as pollinators.

Identification

The spring beauty belongs to the Montiaceae family. It is a type of perennial species that produces its flowers during Spring. Its pink or white petal with dark veins can be used to identify it.

The ripening of the seed capsules usually leads to the vanishing of the plant from above the ground.

Each of the flowers contains six white petals covered by pink veins. A pair of the leaves grow on the stems and a leaf measures about 8cm in length and 2cm in width.

Edible Parts

The roots, leaves, and stems are edible. Their roots are rich in starch and have a nutty flavor.

Safe Consumable Quantity

Eat as much as you desire.

Best Consumable State

The roots, leaves, and stems can be eaten raw or cooked.

Nutritional Value

It's rich in Vitamin A and C.

Location

They are usually found in forests, open woods, wetlands, and in alluvial thickets.

Tea Plant

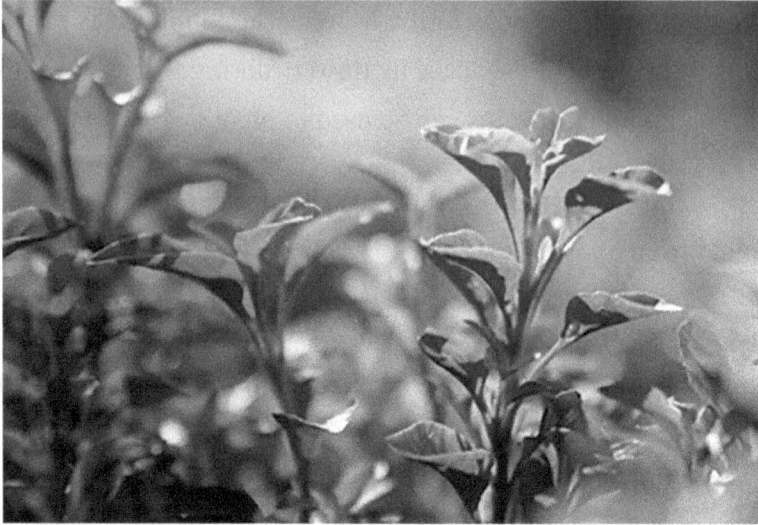

The tea plant is also known as Camellia Sinensis. It is the source of different kinds of teas including, white, yellow, black, and oolong tea.

The tea is produced from the leaf buds and the leaves. What differentiates the tea color from another is in the process of production adopted by the producer.

Identification

It is known as an evergreen shrub but can grow into a tree if left undisturbed. It can last for up to 50 years. Their flowers are always white with a fragrant aroma. They sometimes appear in clusters of between 2 to 4.

Flowers of the plants are hermaphrodite, which are pollinated by bees. The leaves are dark green with a pointed tip. Leaves have a hairy underside and can grow to about 8 cm in length.

They are commonly found in shaded areas with a high elevation at forest edges. It thrives in an area filled with sandy or partially loamy soil.

Edible Parts

The leaves are edible for food or tea. It is advisable to eat it raw if you want to enjoy the nutrients of the leaf fully. Tea flower is also suitable for consumption.

Safe Consumable Quantity

Take it in moderation.

Best Consumable State

Tea leaves can be eaten as food or used in making tea.

Nutritional Value

Tea plants have flavonoids, amino acids, and proteins.

Location

It can be found in warmer parts of North America.

Toothwort

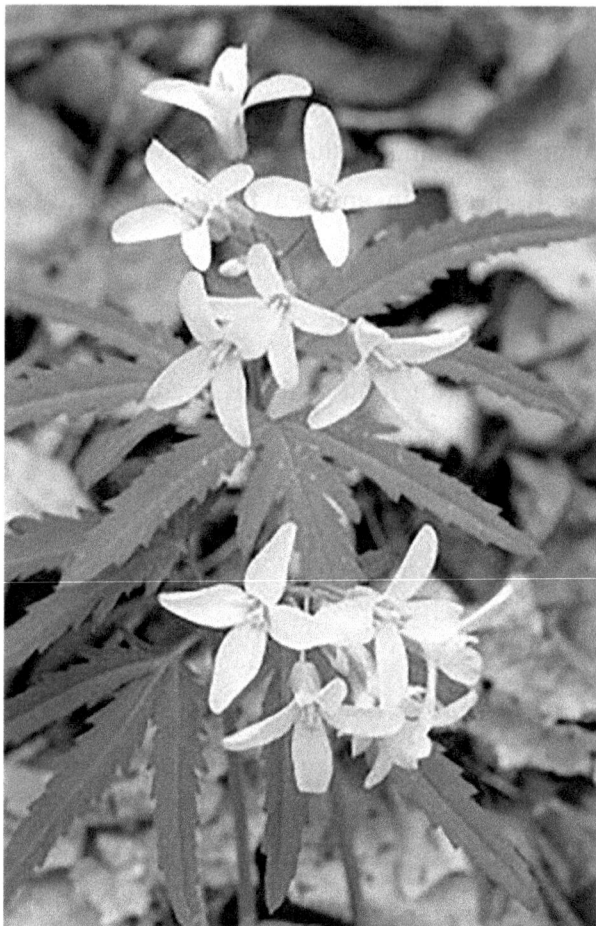

The toothwort, also called the Dentaria diphylla plant, belongs to the Brassicaceae family.

Identification

It grows during the Spring, and it remains as a woodland groundcover through the summer. The plant goes dormant immediately after flowering and returns in the fall. Flowers on the plants thrive within March to April.

Each flower possesses four petals with a white to pinkish color. Toothwort leaves are basal and have a long petiole. Generally, the wild plant can grow to about 30 to 40 cm tall.

Edible Parts

You can add leaves to a salad or slice it into soups. The root of the plant has a pungent taste, especially when it is first harvested. The root will develop a sweet taste if left to be fermented for about three days.

Safe Consumable Quantity

Take it in moderation.

Best Consumable State

Both the leaves and the roots of the plants can be eaten raw or cooked.

Location

The toothwort plant is native to North America. They are usually found in the northeast of the U.S., Ontario, and down to the Maritimes in Canada. The plant mostly grows in woods and meadows with moist soils.

Teasel

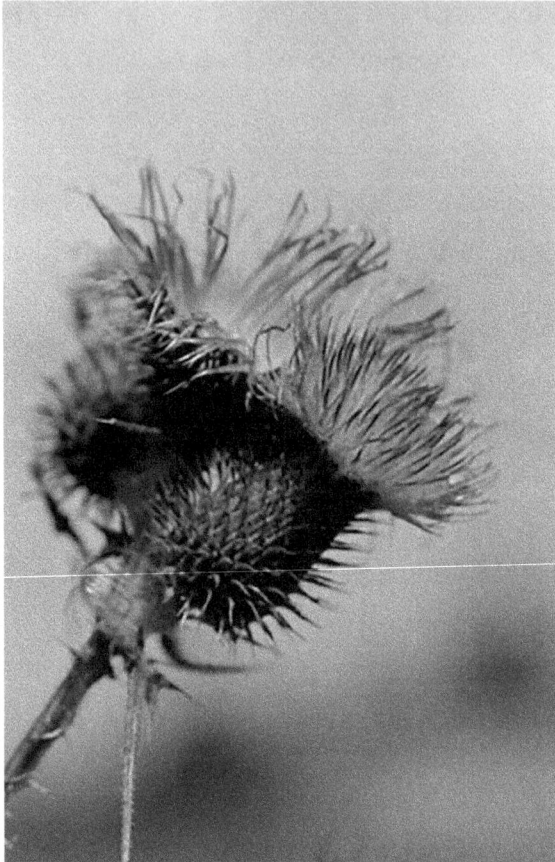

Teasel is also known as Dipsacus fullonum. It is a biennial plant that can be easily identified. The plant is self-fertile, and it is known to attract wildlife. The first year of the plant produces a set of rosette leaves and grows to about 2.5 meters in the following year.

Identification

You can identify Teasel by its thick taproot and fibrous secondary roots. After the first year, the flower forms a ring in the middle of its head. It then grows for a few days before it withers, leaving two rings growing in opposite directions.

The whole flower head measures about 50 to 100 cm in height with a single flower measuring approximately 12 mm.

Flowers are lilac in color and grows on the plant between June and September. Flowering stems usually stands upright and branches close to the top of the plant.

Edible Parts
The leaves and roots are edible.

Safe Consumable Quantity
Eat as you deem fit.

Best Consumable State
You can choose to eat the leaves raw, cooked, or even add it to a smoothie. The roots can be used to make vinegar or tea.

Nutritional Value
It's rich in fiber, vitamin C, and flavonoids.

Location
Teasels can be found in many parts of the world in sunny areas. It can be found in roadsides, pastures, abandoned fields, and wastelands.

Wild Grape Vines

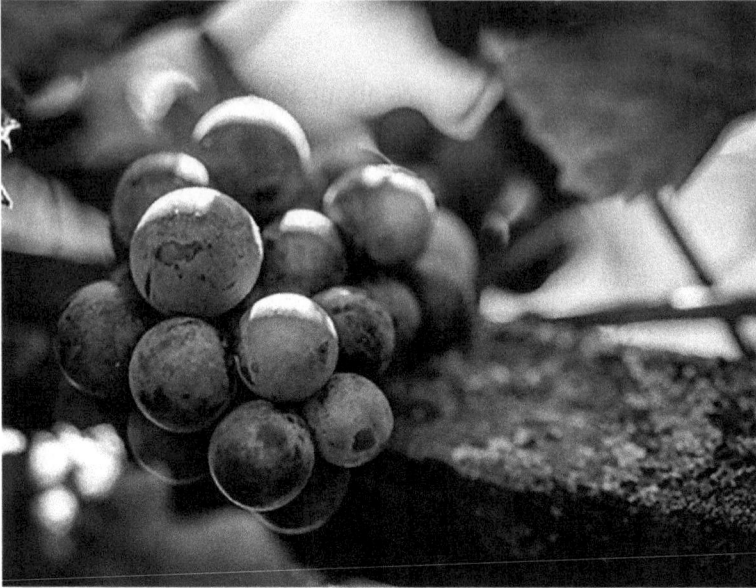

Wild grapes, also called Vitis Riparia, are deciduous vines with a voracious growth pattern. Its growth can overshadow other trees or bushes around.

Dozens of this plant grow across different areas of the world. They are perennial plants that grow well above other native vines.

Identification

Grapevines usually produce deep-lobed leaves which are similar to a cultivated grape. It climbs very well during its growth because of its forking tendrils. They are generally purple, black, or dark blue. Tiny flowers of about 10 cm in length grows on the plant.

The flowers bloom early in summer before green grapes start to develop. The leaves alternate along the stem and can grow to about

15 cm in length. They are orbicular in shape and are faintly or deeply lobed.

The edges are well toothed with hairy texture. Generally, wild grapes can grow to about 17 meters in length.

Edible Parts

Wild grape tastes better after the initial frost, but you can also eat the ripe grapes. You will thoroughly enjoy the grape when you make it into juice.

Safe Consumable Quantity

Eat it in moderation. It could add up to the carbs and calories in your body quickly.

Best Consumable State

The leaves can also be eaten raw or added to a salad. The fruit can also be eaten raw.

Nutritional Value

They are a rich source of vitamin A, C, carbohydrates, and protein.

Location

You'll find up to 60 species of this plant in North America.

Wild Bee Balm

Wild bee balm is also known as wild bergamot. It is an aromatic plant that attracts bees, birds, and butterflies. Native Americans commonly use it as a cure for the common cold.

Wild bee balm grows from creeping rhizomes.

Identification

Wild bee plants can be easily identified from other plants by its rough lavender or pink color. The plant shows resistance to drought and only thrives in sunny and dry areas. Monarda didyma shares similar characteristics with the wild bee plant and can be differentiated by its red color.

The flowers are fragrant and bloom from the center of the flower head down to the periphery. It blooms for around one month, starting from mid-summer. Alternate leaves are ovate or lanceolate and usually vary in color.

Environmental conditions will determine whether the leaves will turn out light or dark green. Wild bee balm generally grows to about 30 to 70 cm tall in their lifetime.

Edible Parts

They are usually used as flavors in cooked foods or salads. Wild bee balm's flower can also be used to garnish salads.

Safe Consumable Quantity

It's okay to eat it moderation, but pregnant women should avoid it.

Best Consumable State

The leaves can be eaten raw or cooked.

Nutritional Value

It contains caffeic acid.

Location

The plants are generally seen in borders of limestone glades, fields, and thickets.

Vervain Mallow

Vervain mallow was initially known to be a cultivated plant, but it now grows well in the wild. It is a natural source for green, yellow and cream-colored dyes.

They generally thrive in areas with a balanced pH or alkaline-rich areas.

Identification

Its delicate flower texture can make it easy to identify. The flowers bloom, irrespective of the weather conditions at any particular time. This perennial plant can grow to more than 50 cm in height. The flowers contain five white or pink petals and five green sepals.

The flower is about 3 to 9 cm in width, with the petals measuring the length of the sepal thrice. Vervain mallow leaves possess long petioles with about 3 to 8 cm in length. The top of the leaves is usually dark green in color and light green underneath.

Edible Parts

The seed, flowers, and leaves of Vervain mallow are all edible. The seeds are the tastiest part of the plant.

Safe Consumable Quantity

It's best to eat in moderate quantities.

Best Consumable State

The leaves are relatively bland and can be eaten raw or cooked.

Nutritional Value

The plants are dense in vitamin E, C, and magnesium.

Location

It's a common plant in North America. They usually grow in wastelands or thickets.

Prickly Pear Cactus

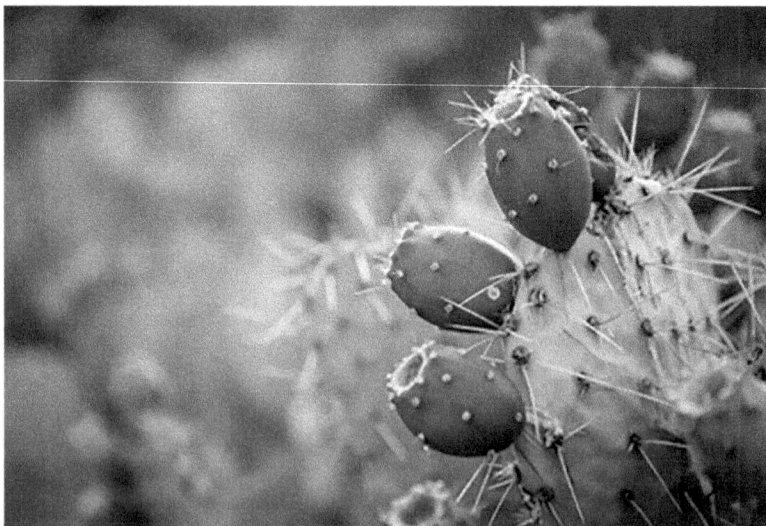

The origin of prickly pear cactus can be traced back to South America before migrating to Mexico and the southern U.S. It depicts fifteen other species of the Opuntia genus across North America.

Identification

They are perennial plants and are often characterized by fleshy, jointed, and flattened stem-segments called the pads. The pads are modified stems or branches that perform different functions in the plant. They are responsible for storing water, flower production, and photosynthesis as well.

Their flowers usually bloom from around April to June. Depending on the species, some can be yellow, peach, orange, cream, or any combination of those colors. They do not have leaves. Prickly pears roughly grow to about 1.5 meters and can spread to about 4.5 meters in diameter.

Edible Parts

Both the fruits and pads are suitable for consumption. The edible prickly pears are those with pads that look like beavers' tail. The cholla cacti species, which are known by their slender and rounded stems, are not edible.

Safe Consumable Quantity

Too much of it can cause nausea, abdominal pain in some people.

Best Consumable State

You can consume its fruits fresh.

Nutritional Value

It's rich in carbohydrate, protein, vitamin A & C, calcium, and phosphorus.

Location

Most species of prickly pear are native to North America.

Herb Robert

Herb Robert was named after a French monk who used the plant to cure many folks suffering from different diseases. It is widely known in the 1000 AD as a potent cure for internal and external ailments.

According to research, scientists discovered that the plant thrives in areas with high radiation. From the study, it is believed that the plant absorbs radiation from the ground and disperses it around.

Identification

You can quickly identify the plant by its unpleasant smell and its bright pink color. The flower blossoms from Spring down to October. The flower is radial star-shaped and measures between 1.5 to 2 cm across its end. It contains five petals that are round-tipped with paler veins. You will see up to ten stamens on the flower, and the pistil contains five carpels.

The leaves contain partially dark green colors of about 6cm, with the edges having purple colors. The plant is known to grow abundant leaves, even if the plants are picked regularly. Herb Robert usually grows to about 30 to 40 cm in their lifetime.

Edible Parts

Both the flower and the leaves are safe for consumption. They can be dried and stored to be used throughout the winter. Rubbing the fresh leaves on the skin can help repel mosquitoes.

Safe Consumable Quantity

Eat as you deem fit.

Best Consumable State

It can be added to diets raw or fresh.

Nutritional Value

It's rich in Vitamins A and C, and carotenoids.

Location

It's common in most parts of North America.

Mayapple

This perennial plant belongs to the Barberry family. Its uniqueness stems from its two umbrella-like leaves with one flower after maturity. You can easily spot the plant from afar because its rhizomes form dense mats. It usually survives in moist and humus-rich soils.

Identification

Mayapple is one of the few plants to grow from the ground during Spring. Its big, deeply cut leaves can quickly identify it. A flower usually forms below the leaves and later transforms into a yellow fruit.

The flowers develop from the axil of the leaves with 6 to 9 petals. Yellow stamens surround its large greenish-yellow ovary.

The mayapple leaves are conspicuous because of their large umbrella-like leaves. As the stem lengthens out, the leaves remain closed and later unfolds to about 15 cm across. The leaves keep on growing until it reaches a total length of about 40 cm across. Generally, mayapples grow to about 30 – 40 cm high with stout and smooth stem.

Edible Parts

The only edible part of the mayapple is the yellow fruit. The seed must be removed before eating. Make sure the fruit has changed to yellow before consuming because unripe ones are not safe for consumption. You can also use the fruit to make smoothies.

Safe Consumable Quantity

Overeating it may cause colic. You should only eat a moderate quantity.

Best Consumable State

Only the ripe yellow fruit can be eaten.

Location

It is commonly found across North America.

Joe Pye Weed

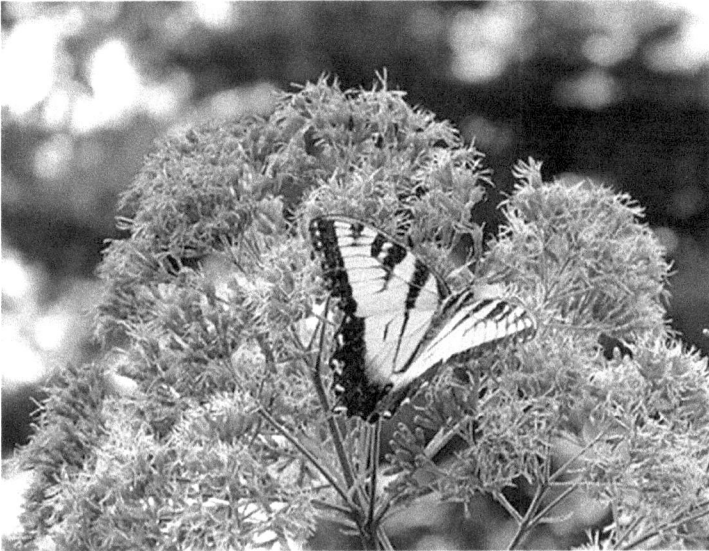

Joe Pye weed serves as a multipurpose wild plant. It is used as an herb, butterfly plants and also cultivated in some places as flower beds.

People believe the plant's name originates from a Native American named Joe Pye (Jopi). He used the plant as a cure for typhus in the 19th century. It is a perennial plant that blooms after other plants have stopped.

Identification

You can identify the plant by its pink or purple-colored flowers at the end of its stem. The flowers sprout at the stems from around July to late fall. They have a large flower head with a domed cluster of pink disk flowers.

The leaves form a concentric circle and can grow to about 25 cm in height. Each node contains four to seven blades, and the leaves are elliptical. Generally, Joe Pye weed can grow to about 1 meter in length. They are mostly found in marshes, moist woods, damp thickets, along streams, and fields.

Edible Parts

Any part of the plant can be eaten, including the root. You can dry the leaves and stems for later use. The fresh flowers can be used to make herbal tea.

Safe Consumable Quantity

It is best to eat in moderate quantities.

Best Consumable State

It is best consumed fresh or dried for later use.

Location

The plant is native to North America.

Knapweed

The botanical name for Knapweed is called Centaurea nigra, and it is also referred to as Hardheads. The Knapweed can last for years as a neglected grassland or as a grazed pasture. Insects like flies, bees, beetles, and butterflies pollinate its flowers.

Identification

The Knapweed thrives in areas with low or moderately fertile soil. You can identify the plant by its dull green color, which is covered by rough hairs. They have erect stems which are branched at the top.

Knapweed's flower heads grow at the branch tips with the base covered with dark fringed margins. The flower generally sprouts from June to September, depending on the location.

The leaves are alternate and are pale green. Lower leaves on the plant are sometimes toothed and may grow to about 25 cm in length. Generally, the Knapweed grows to about 1 meter in length in its lifetime. They can be found in meadows, pastures, field borders, woodland edges, and roadsides.

Edible Parts
Knapweed is generally used for medicinal purposes. Only the flowers are safe for consumption.

Safe Consumable Quantity
Eat as you deem fit.

Best Consumable State
You can eat it raw or cooked, depending on your preference.

Nutritional Value
It is rich in carbohydrate, protein, fiber, and Ash.

Location
It is commonly found in Canada and some other parts of North America.

Wild Leek

Wild leeks belong to the same family as onion, and it is one of the earliest edible wild plants that appear during springs. It is widely used in the past as a spring tonic for restoration after a prolonged winter.

Two varieties of wild leek exist, namely, Var. tricoccum and Var. burdickii. The former is characterized by a red base and a cluster of around 50 flowers. The latter has narrow leaves with about 20 clusters.

Identification

Wild leeks feature an elliptical-shaped leaf that usually comes up in the Spring. You can quickly identify them by their scent, which is similar to that of onions. You might need to crush its leaf to tell the difference through the onion scent correctly.

The flowers grow after the leaves have emerged for like four weeks. The white flower produced has six petals and six stamens with a creamy yellow tip.

The leaves grow from an underground bulb during the early springs. They grow to about 15 to 30 cm in length and 2 to 10 cm in width. It features a smooth texture with parallel veins. Generally, Wild leeks grow to about 45 cm in length and are mostly found in forests.

Edible Parts

The leaves and the bulbs are edible. It is advisable to take one leaf per plant because of its seven years growth cycle.

Safe Consumable Quantity

Eat as you deem fit.

Best Consumable State

The leaves and the bulbs can either be eaten raw or cooked.

Nutritional Value

It is rich in vitamins and minerals.

Location

It can be found in many parts of North America.

Cleavers

The cleavers belongs to the Rubiaceae family. More than 3000 species exist in the Rubiaceae family. People call the plant other names like a sticky bud, sticky willy, kisses, stickyweed, and clivers.

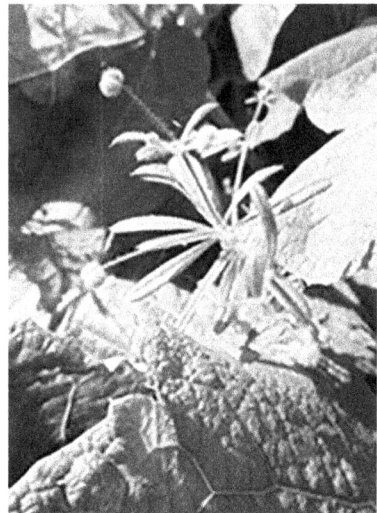

Identification

Cleavers are an annual plant that creeps with spreading stems. They grow by attaching themselves to anything on their way with hooked hairs. The flowers are tiny, measuring about 1mm in length and 1 to 2 mm in width. They are white with four petals joined together at the base.

Two distinct types of leaves grow on Cleavers, namely, stalkless leaves and cleaver leaves. The stalkless leaves grow in a group of 6 to 9 at the stem joint.

The cleaver leaves are narrow with pointed tips. They do not grow in height, except they attach themselves to a tall plant. Cleavers are commonly found in field margins and hedgerows.

Edible Parts

The leaves and the stems are both safe for consumption. They are also used in the past for medicinal purposes. The fruit can be dried and used as a coffee substitute. Some folks also dry the leaves for tea.

Safe Consumable Quantity

You can eat as you deem it fit. For those who feel rash after touching the plants, don't eat it at all.

Best Consumable State

The leaves and stem can be eaten raw or cooked. You can also use it in sandwiches.

Location

It is mostly found in North America, Europe, and Asia.

Cattail

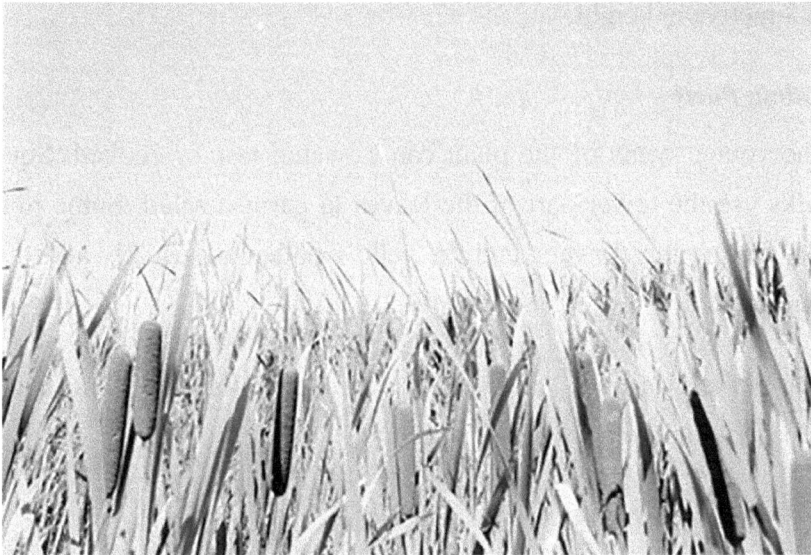

Cattails are also known as bulrushes, and they are among the most common wild foods. They are usually used in making mats and baskets. The Aboriginals use the plant as a source of flour.

Identification

Cattails can easily be identified by its cigar-shaped head, which is brown. During springs, the young shoots grow and later transforms into a cigar-like head. This cigar contains thousands of developing seeds in them.

The flowers are made up of the male and female cigar-like formation. The male part is the yellow spike that rises above the female part.

Cattail leaves are erect, linear, flat, and dome-shaped, measuring between 10 mm to 20 mm in width. Each vegetative shoot produces between 12 to 16 leaves. Cattails stand upright, averaging around 2 to 3 meters in height.

Edible Parts

The young stems of the plant can be eaten raw or cooked. Some folks use the lower part of the leaves to garnish salad. Some roast the blossoming flowers, and the yellow pollen are usually added to pancakes.

The pollens can also be used as a thickener for stews and soups after shaking them well in a paper bag.

Safe Consumable Quantity

Eat as you deem fit.

Best Consumable State

Go for the younger edible parts, and consume them raw or cooked.

Nutritional Value

It is rich in carbohydrates and protein.

Location

They thrive in swamps, open wet areas, moist fields, and ditches.

Blue Vervain

The Blue Vervain belongs to the Verbenaceae family. Apart from being a wild plant, it has become one of the top choices for landscaped gardens. It is a perennial plant that is often pollinated by bees.

Identification

You can identify the Blue Vervain from its 4-angled stems, which sometimes have white hairs. It is a tall and upright plant that branches above its midpoint. Blooming usually takes place around late Spring down to late summer, depending on the geographic location.

The wildflower is made up of many pencil-like tips that branch upward. A ring of purple flowers is arrayed on each flower. The leaves of Blue Vervain are aligned opposite to one another with length ranging from 3cm to 17cm.

Dark green color with strong veins characterizes them. Blue Vervain generally grows between 30 cm to around 2 meters in their lifetime.

Edible Parts

It is safe to consume the seed, flower, and leaves. You can only eat the grounded and the roasted form of the seed. The flowers and the leaves can be tossed into a salad to garnish it. It is also known for its medicinal use by medical herbalists.

Safe Consumable Quantity

It can be eaten as much as you desire. People with kidney diseases should avoid eating this plant.

Best Consumable State

The leaves and flowers can be eaten raw or cooked. The seed can only be eaten after grounding or roasting it.

Location

It is a common plant across the U.S. and Canada. It thrives on moist areas with little exposure to the sun.

Common Yarrow

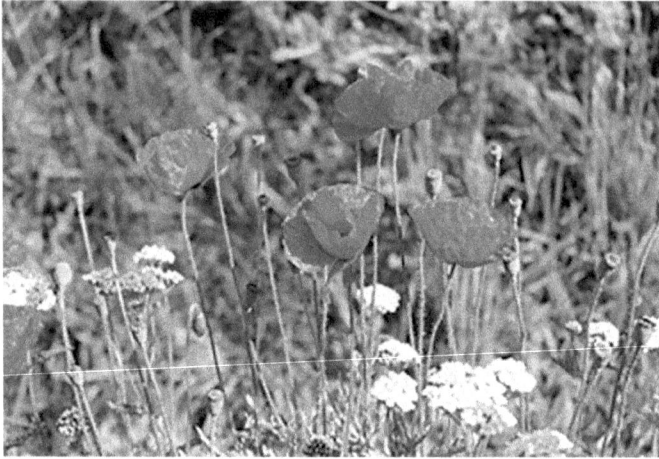

The Common Yarrow is also known as Achillea millefolium. It is a perennial wild plant that is often referred to as an aggressive weed.

The name Achillea was adopted from Achilles in the Trojan wars, who used it to heal his soldier's wounds.

Identification

Its aromatic and fern-like green foliage can identify Common Yarrow. They are made up of tiny dense flowers that flattens out. It is a common plant that grows in both the wild and gardens too. The flower heads grow on the stem in clusters with each cluster containing at least one flower head. Each flower head contains about 20 to 25 white ray flowers.

Leaves of this plant span to about 7 to 12 cm in length. Each midrib contains many leaflets on either side, which are also subdivided into smaller leaflets. Generally, the Yarrow plant usually grows between 30 cm to 1 meter.

Edible Parts

The flowers and leaves are edible. They can be used to make tea. Adding the leaves to a salad can also be a great combination.

Safe Consumable Quantity

Moderate or little quantity should be used per time.

Best Consumable State

The leaves of this wild plant can be consumed raw or cooked and are best eaten when it is still young.

Location

It is a common plant that is usually found in most parts of North America. They thrive in sunny areas with sandy soils.

Common Sow Thistle

The common sow thistle belongs to the Compositae family. It is often eaten because of its wide range of minerals.

Identification

You can quickly identify them by their hollow stems that eject latex when broken. The taproot is short, and the leaves are lobed. The flowers are yellow, with a diameter of about 5 to 6 mm. You will find the flowers at the plant's stalk near its branch end.

The first set of leaves are round and has a toothed margin. Hairs are dotted on the surface of the leaves, and the mature leaves are thinner. The mature leaves are dark green with an irregularly toothed margin. The plant grows to about 30cm to 1m in height. The plant thrives on most soil types and can be found in yards, pastures, fields, and so on.

Edible Parts

The flowers, leaves, and young roots of this plant are edible.

Safe Consumable Quantity

Eat as you deem fit.

Best Consumable State

The plant tastes best in its early season. Flowers and leaves can be tossed into a salad or cooked with spinach and soups. You can prepare the young roots and the stems as well.

Nutritional Value

It is rich in minerals like magnesium, calcium, potassium, sodium, iron phosphorus, zinc, and vitamins.

Location

Though native to Europe, it grows in many parts of North America.

Coltsfoot

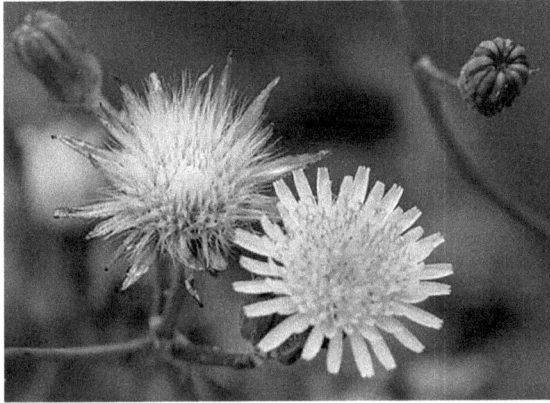

Coltsfoot is a perennial plant that is generally called "son before the father." It earns this name because the flowers grow and die before the leaves appear. It looks like a dandelion when the plant blooms in the Spring. Some people use it for the treatment and prevention of cough.

Identification

Its bright yellow flowers can be used to identify it as it blooms during early Spring. The flowers are single, with an average width of about 1.5 cm. Many pistillate flowers and ray florets are arranged on the flowers with white stamens.

The surface of the leaf is smooth and waxy in appearance. The leaves are dotted with white hairs underneath. The average height of Coltsfoot is about 10 to 15 cm.

Edible Parts

The flowers and the leaves are both safe for consumption.

Safe Consumable Quantity

It is advisable to use moderate quantity because the leaves have a somewhat bitter taste.

Best Consumable State

You can also add the edible parts into salads. Adding the flower with honey has been proven to help subside cough. The leaves have a somewhat bitter taste, and it is advisable to boil before adding to a soup.

Location

It thrives on open areas and is commonly found in roadsides, ditches, forest edges, and landslides.

Fern Leaf Yarrow

The Fern Leaf Yarrow is also known as Achillea filipendulina. It is famous for its antiseptic and anti-inflammatory use.

It contains many minerals and vitamins that are beneficial to your health. It is also used for treating colds, kidney diseases, menstrual pain, wounds, and many more.

Identification

You can identify this wild plant by its single stout stem. Disk flowers and tiny rays grow on this stem. The flowers are yellow, and they grow in large clusters called compound corymb. The corymbs are usually up to 10 cm across.

The leaves measure between 5 to 20 cm in length. They grow almost evenly in a curly manner on the stem.

Edible Parts

The young leaves are recommended for salads. It is often used as a preservative for beer.

Safe Consumable Quantity

Though nutritious, it is advisable not to consume the plant regularly.

Best Consumable State

The leaves are bitter and can be eaten raw or cooked.

Location

It is common in North America as well as in many parts of the world. They are usually found in the countryside, waste areas, along the highways, meadows, and pastures.

Final Words

Knowing everything on a wild plant will help foragers to understand what works best in every season. Most of these wild plants are located within your vicinity. You can decide to add some to your landscape for easy accessibility. No matter whether you are new to foraging, or you are a pro, there is always a plant for you to find.

It is not enough to just find these plants, though. You need to know the right way to harvest and store them. You will learn all about that in the next chapter.

Chapter 7

Harvesting and Storage Tips for Wild Edible Plants

Harvesting and storage are two of the essential parts of foraging. Harvesting involves all the processes that include bringing proceeds back from the field. Storage refers to all processes involved in ensuring continued use of the harvested proceeds.

The demand for wild edible plants has been on the rise recently. This rise in demand is due to the increased awareness of health and wellbeing.

Many restaurants have started to add wild species to their menu. Just like many healthy food options out there, it doesn't come cheap. Restaurants pay handsomely for these wild species.

Most restaurants would pay more to have their plants delivered fresh. Unfortunately, most of these species are perishable. Invariably, you have to make sure your plants are delivered fresh.

Some of these species are also seasonal. Demand, on the other hand, is not seasonal. Finding a way to keep them against scarcity gives you some advantage in price.

Therefore, harvesting and storage go hand in hand.

Even if you are keeping them for personal reasons, storage is still vital. The process involved in foraging could be stressful. Storage helps you save some for later use. That way, you don't have to go out every time in search of wild plants.

Tips for Harvesting Wild plants

Harvesting wild plants can be a lot of fun. It can also become a catastrophe, especially if you are a novice. The problem here is you might even be doing something wrong unknowingly. Therefore, even as a veteran, you would find the following harvesting tips helpful.

1. Gather Information on Identification

This step should not be skipped. It is crucial because some plants are dangerous to consume. Some of these dangerous plants are similar to the edible species. Some plant families are not consumable across the board. You might find many similar relatives while harvesting.

Ensure you get proper education to avoid picking potentially dangerous plants. Get familiar with your plants before going to the field.

While some plants are dangerous to consume, some are deadly to touch. Severe allergic reactions could result from merely touching some species.

You should know what to avoid before going to the field. More importantly, you should understand why you need to avoid them.

2. Understand the Area

Before you go out to harvest, you should know the area. Your ideal harvest spot should be free of pollutants. Pollutants could be in the form of herbicides or insecticides. The place should also be free from toxic wastes.

Also, check the growth conditions of the plants. Do not pick plants that are struggling to grow. For instance, you should not choose plants growing under drought or poor soil fertility.

More importantly, only harvest from areas where you are permitted. Also, try to change the harvest location as often as you can.

3. Understand the Plant

Understanding the plant comes in different forms. You should also learn how best to harvest the plants without killing them. That way, the plants can be useful for as long as you need them.

In understanding your plants, you should know the best time to harvest them. Different plants have different seasons when they are at their best. Also, their parts do well at different times of the year. Do a little research to know when it's best to harvest what you need.

4. Harvest What You Need Alone

Thinking about seasonality, you might be tempted to take a little too much. It is wrong on several levels.

Firstly, you could be putting the species in danger of extinction. If you continue harvesting so much, you might harvest all there is to harvest of such species.

Secondly, taking too much at a time could result in wastage. You might take so much that you wouldn't be able to store. Eventually, it gets wasted.

You should have an idea of how much you need to avoid having waste. With proper storage, you could store some species for six months. This period is longer than the offseason for most wild species. So, your estimates should project how much you would need for that long.

You should only take about 5% of the population of a particular species. Your harvest spot should have such species in abundance.

Keep in mind that you are not the only person harvesting. Therefore, harvest in a manner that leaves a lot behind for others.

5. After Harvest

After harvesting your plants, you should think of the future. If the opportunity presents itself, replace the plants with their seeds. That way, you would have something to fall back to in the future.

Tips for Storing Wild Plants

The following tips will help you keep your harvest and retain its freshness.

1. Keep Your Plants Dry

While collecting your plants, it is possible to pick them with water. You could have dew on them, especially if you harvest in the morning. Ensure you remove the water droplets to keep them for long in storage.

2. Keep Separately

Keep different species differently. This approach will prevent contamination.

Also, keep different plant parts separated from one another when you need to. For instance, if you would be collecting flowers and roots, the roots should be kept away from the flowers. As you would know, the roots would come with dirt, which can affect the flowers.

Keep green parts in paper bags alternatively. You could use containers that allow them to breathe. Whichever you choose, try not to overfill.

3. Refresh Before Storing

Right after you leave the field, try to refresh your plants before storing them. Restoring them involves rinsing them in cold water. This practice would keep them fresh and clean for as long as you would need them.

4. Refrigerate as Soon as You Can

Immediately you return from the field, refrigerate your greens. Also, sort out other parts that need refrigeration and do the same. This habit would help them retain their freshness and prevent wilting.

Sometimes, the distance from the harvest point to the field might be far. Consider going along with cooling units if you can.

5. Avoid Using Plastic

Plastic raises the temperature, no matter how careful you are. Increased temperature will always have adverse impacts on the storage of your plants. As much as you can, find healthy alternatives to plastics.

Final Words

Harvesting and storage are essential parts of foraging for wild plants. Most times, the two processes go hand in hand. Both methods aim to have safe plants for continued consumption.

Safety is crucial in foraging. We have provided some tips that you need to take note of when you go foraging.

Chapter 8

Tips on Foraging

Foraging is an exciting experience, but it can also be wrongly done. It all boils down to playing by the rules. Luckily, these rules or tips are not hard to comply with. Getting this book is a step in the right direction.

The tips below will guide you whenever you forage. These are simple tips you should know before, during, and after foraging.

General Tips for Foraging

There are certain things you need to know about foraging before you go out. We have provided these tips to help you on your journey.

Know Your Region

It is essential to understand the region in which you would be foraging. Do proper research on the landscape of the area where you intend to forage.

Emissions from mines or other industrial structures could contaminate the water or soil that nourishes the plant you intend to forage. These contaminants could make you fall sick.

Mushrooms absorb pollutants quickly. Avoid picking mushrooms close to industrial areas or busy roads.

Also, the kinds of herbicides, pesticides, or other chemicals used can affect the plants and affect you indirectly. Therefore, ensure you do your research.

This process involves in-depth research on the terrain. Online courses and eBooks, just like one, are great places to start.

Knowing your region helps you know the type of plants that are cultivated there. This knowledge brings us to the second point.

Know Your Plants

Foraging includes wild plants that can be extremely poisonous. Therefore, you should be able to differentiate between edible plants and those that are not edible. A little mistake can be costly. Some plants can have terrible effects on your health.

For example, giant hogweed, iris, poison hemlock, monkshood are common wild plants found in North America. These plants are not suitable for food. So, if you would be foraging in North America, you have to be able to identify these plants and avoid them.

Plants like cattails, pine, and mint are safe and edible, regardless of the location. Some additional tips that will help you are;

- It is advisable to forage with an expert - someone who can correctly identify these plants.

- When in doubt, stick with what you know. You can explore the regular plants that you are familiar with.

- The rule of thumb for foragers is if you cannot identify it, do not eat it.

- It is advisable to move from the known edible plants to the unknown. However, in extreme cases of starvation, ensure you test first time plants before consuming.

Tips to Test Plant Edibility

- Divide the plant into different parts- stems, leaves, etc. then test separately.

- Discard plant parts or secretions, such as sap that have a bad odor or taste.

- Touch your skin with a small part of the plant and wait for ten minutes. This action helps you test for contact poisoning. If you get any reaction such as rashes, inflammation, etc., do not eat the plant.

- If there is no reaction, touch a small part of the plant on your lips. Wait for another ten minutes.

- Then, use your tongue to taste the plant. Wait for ten minutes too.

- If there is no reaction, eat a small part of the plant. Wait for about 7-10 hours

- If you feel like you are getting ill, try to induce vomiting. Then, do not eat the plant.

- If you feel good after these steps, you are good to go.

Do not forget that you should only use these tips in extreme cases. Correctly identifying your plants and your area comes first.

Also, these tips may not be very efficient for mushrooms. Some mushrooms taste so great, but they are entirely poisonous. You have to be extra careful with mushrooms.

You can check the internet for a list of dangerous plants in your area and how to identify them. Books or guides are good companions when foraging. Books that contain pictures of edible and poisonous plants are good sources of knowledge.

If in doubt, don't eat it!

Ask Questions

Ask the natives in the area (if there are natives present). These natives know more about the plants than you do. You can get some information about the land and plants. They could serve as your foraging guide. Some tips that you should take into are;

- Plants that are safe for animals are not automatically safe for humans. Do not make this assumption.

- Do not test two new plants at the same time. Try one new plant after the order.

- Clean your plants very well. Mushrooms have to be thoroughly clean because they have accumulated manure, and it could have remnants of fungi or bacteria. Berries, on the other hand, has to be cleaned under a gentle flow of water. Use clean water when washing your plants.

- When foraging with your family, ensure you keep an eye on your kids. Do not let them eat any plants on their own.

- Stay away from plants that are grown by the roadside. If you must eat plants grown by the roadside, ensure that you wash them thoroughly to avoid contamination.

- Not all plants should be eaten raw. Some kinds of mushrooms are poisonous when eaten fresh. You would have to boil some and cook others. Check up on ways to safely prepare wild plants. Also, liver flukes are found in wet plants in their larval stage, and they can cause severe health problems. These problems can be averted by cooking or boiling the plants.

- Different wild plants and mushrooms grow in different seasons. It is advisable to look up plants and their seasons to know what to expect when foraging. Some types of mushrooms grow at certain times of the year. For example, fruits such as acorn, blackberries, and chestnuts are found in abundance during winter.

Know Yourself

You must have a list of your allergies and food sensitivities. Avoid plants that can trigger your allergies. Because it is good for your friend does not mean that it is good for you.

- When in doubt as to whether you are allergic to a particular plant, practice the edibility test described above.

- Avoid wild plants or mushrooms when you are pregnant. Wild plants and mushrooms can contain chemicals that can hurt your baby. For example, some kinds of pine needles can cause miscarriages.

Tips To Consider During Foraging

- Do not take more than you can consume to avoid wastage.

- When harvesting plants, be careful so as not to cause damage to your plants. Harvest with care. Pick berries with utmost care.

- Harvest from species that are densely populated. Take mushrooms that have their caps opened already. They have shed their spores so they can reproduce.

- Every forager should be conscious of the ecosystem. Foraging activities can sometimes disrupt the ecosystem. It is advised that you start with weeds to avoid this problem. Some plants grow almost immediately after harvest.

Plantain and nettle are examples of weeds that multiply quickly and are safe.

- Do not harvest all the plants. For the sake of preservation and the ecosystem, always leave some plants behind. Some birds and other animals feed on these plants. Also, remember that others forage too. Some of these plants need to be replaced. They need to produce seed and spores for another cycle of growth. It aids continuity and balance.

- The law protects some wild plants, especially rare plants. Ensure you know the plants that you are allowed to forage. You can also take a field guide when foraging to help.

- Ensure you have gotten permission from the owner of the land. The owners could be the natives or the government. You do not want to harvest plants on private property or government land.

- Keep a record of new plants, new locations, or any other information when you discover them. It will serve as your guide when you go foraging in the future.

- Clean your environment after every forage exercise.

- Never go foraging in an unknown area all by yourself. Go in groups, with natives or with an expert.

Tips for Forage Clothing

- Light and comfortable clothing are the best choices for foraging. A pair of jeans, a long sleeve shirt, and comfortable running shoes or hiking boots are perfect for hiking.

- You would need to protect your skin from insect infestation. You can also travel with insect repellant. Ensure you are well covered from head to toe. Wear socks if you may.

- Some examples of supplies or equipment that would come in handy include scissors, paper, and cloth bags, a sharp knife, and a trowel all in a convenient bag pack.

- Ensure you do not overload yourself with too many unnecessary items.

Additional Tips for Foraging during Hiking Activities

It is not uncommon to see people combining foraging and hiking activities. They go hand in hand in most cases. These tips should be practiced in addition to the instructions above.

- Sometimes, these plants may not sustain you on your trip. You would need a supply of healthy fats and proteins for your journey. So, it is essential to augment feeding with a minimalist diet. Get yourself some nuts or other healthy sources. Remember, it is a minimalist diet, so don't overfeed.

- Fishes are a good source of protein. You can go along with your fish equipment when foraging.

- Go foraging with your knife. Knives help you harvest plants that need to be dug up.

These tips will help keep you safe when you go foraging. Therefore, you must follow them as you forage. You might be concerned, wondering if foraging is worth the time with all the numerous tips that you have to follow.

In the next chapter, you will learn all about the benefits of foraging. We will also help you take a look at the hazards and how you can overcome them.

Chapter 9

Environmental Benefits
and Hazards of Foraging

F oraging has a lot of benefits on a personal level. It presents a cheap source for getting one's meals. While foraging, you get to handpick your food. If you are lucky, you could find rare species. All these benefits come for free.

The number of edible plants out there in the wild is in multiples of what we have in grocery stores. Transportation logistics limits the collection of some of these plants.

Sometimes, it's economically unwise to collect some species, when compared to the available supply of some species and the harvesting process. On a large scale, it might not be profitable.

However, foraging allows you to taste some of this species. Sometimes, little quantities of these unique tastes could be everything.

While treating yourself to some once in a lifetime flavors, you also get nourishment. Wild species are known to be more nutritious than their domesticated types.

For example, wild dandelions contain about seven times more phytonutrients compared with spinach. Similarly, depending on the variety, wild apples could contain 100 times more phytonutrients compared with those sold at grocery stores.

Besides, you are assured of fresh and uncontaminated food. Since you get to pick your food yourself, you are assured of relative safety.

While picking up fresh and tasty food, you get to see the outside world. You could hike to harvest locations and stretch to pick some fruits. This form of exercise has rewards of its own. You might even find it more rewarding than going to the gym.

Modern society has robbed us of the opportunity of enjoying some things. One of such things is connecting with the environment.

Instead of just watching from a distance, you are involved directly with nature. You can tell natural cycles and reignite your bond with the world. You can tell what season it is by merely looking at some plants. You can also determine what plants would be abundant at such times.

Is there any better way to connect to the environment? Foraging allows you to connect to the environment seamlessly.

The climax of it all is the benefits foraging has on the environment. Foraging is beneficial, no doubt. However, there are concerns that it might have detrimental effects on the environment.

Almost everything with an advantage comes with its disadvantages. Similarly, foraging has its detriments, even on a personal basis. For instance, one could ingest dangerous species. One could also get arrested, and so on.

In this chapter, we will examine the benefits of foraging on the environment. We will also explore the hazards of foraging on the environment.

Benefits of Foraging on the Environment

Foraging is beneficial to the environment. Here are a few ways foraging comes with added benefits for the environment.

1. Sustainability

The sustainability of a species refers to the ability of that species to exist always. For a species to be sustainable, it must be consumed reasonably. Such species must be used without getting them to extinction.

It is essential because extinction does not only affect the species. From a broader perspective, the effects could be much.

Many may argue that not consuming wild plants preserves the species. Speaking rationally, the best way to exhaust something is to consume them. On the contrary, foragers protect the species they consume.

It is so because foraging is done under some form of ethics. Although informal, these ethics ensure the sustainability of the species.

For example, foragers must spread seeds of their plants after harvesting. It would allow the plants to grow again. Also, foragers are only allowed to take only 5% of the total population of a plant species in place.

2. Improved Biodiversity

When done correctly, foraging improves biodiversity. Biodiversity describes how diverse an ecosystem is. That is, how many different species of plants and animals live in a particular environment.

Scientists have said that there are about 80,000 edible plants in the world. As of today, about 95% of what we eat comes from 30 of those plants. It leaves behind over 99% that are under-utilized.

The success of the species that we eat to date is because man depends on them for survival. Take rice as an example. Man enjoys eating rice. Over the years, a lot of effort has been put in rice to ensure that it doesn't go extinct.

Foraging widens the options of plants we can depend on. It gives us more plants that we can be deliberate about protecting. This action means we will as well want to make these plants succeed.

Besides, a recent study claims that a careful collection of plants is healthy for plant populations.

3. Clean Food Production

During regular food production, a lot of chemical inputs are used. Fertilizers are applied to the soil to enhance productivity. Herbicides are applied to kill weeds, and insecticides are used to prevent insect infestation. The list goes on.

The cropping system that we have as of today has a short scope. This system favors only cultivated species as against what it considers weeds. In the end, these weeds are doomed for destruction by any means. In most cases, harmful chemicals are employed.

Some of these chemicals are left behind in the plants we consume. Over time, they build up in the body to cause harm.

On a larger scale, the use of these chemicals has harmful effects on the environment. Using a chemical fertilizer, for instance, might seem harmless. Unfortunately, it could lead to pollution of waterways. It raises the number of greenhouse gasses in the air.

Pesticides and rodenticides kill wildlife. Eventually, these chemicals reduce biodiversity.

Foraging gives you a rather clean alternative to conventional agriculture. Forage plants grow naturally, leaving out the need for chemicals that could affect the environment.

Foraging also gives an alternative to our monotonous cropping systems. With foraging, many of those species we call weeds can be consumed.

The truth is, some of these 'weeds' are even more nutritious than cultivated plants. With foraging, it's more of a win-win situation. You get nourished from consuming some of the 'weeds.' You also get to control their population, so they do not affect your crops.

As you forage, you are assured of personal safety. You are assured of the safety of the environment, as well.

4. Creation of New Habitats

The species that we now call domesticated where once in the wild. Long before man understood the cultivation of these species, they collected from the wild.

Man learned how to reproduce these plants without having to collect them every time. This evolution meant that man had to take the seedlings of these plants from the wild.

Sometimes, it results in the introduction of some other unwanted plants. This accidental introduction creates new ecosystems that are unique.

5. Appreciation of Nature

Foraging allows people to connect with their environment. They can appreciate the environment and be more concerned about it by doing so.

Foraging helps people understand the seasons. You are intimated with food cycles, meaning that you have to wait for some seasons to enjoy some foods. This lifestyle is a bit different from what you are used to right now. It sort of helps you respect the environment.

More importantly, foraging teaches you about the environment. You get to learn the best ways to harvest your plants and methods of harvesting that encourage sustainability. You will also learn about endangered species.

This way, you can contribute your quota to conservation and preservation.

Hazards of Foraging on the Environment

The hazard of foraging on the environment is a controversial topic. Scientists who are pro-forage believe it's almost harmless. On the other hand, some are of them think that it is dangerous.

The truth, however, sits in between. Foraging, despite its numerous benefits to the environment, can pose just as many risks, especially when the forager is not experienced or deliberately goes against instructions.

The following are instances where foraging could pose a danger to the environment.

1. Overharvesting

One of the significant risks that foraging pose to the environment is overharvesting. Let's face it. Humans would always be humans. There would be the urge to go back for more.

Having in mind that many of these species are highly-priced. People would want to harvest more, harvesting at levels that the environment might not recover from soon. Although some scientists believe this harvesting helps the species.

Also, some scientists believe the population of wild plants out there cannot support everyone. If everyone were to go into foraging, there could be a severe overharvesting problem.

Overharvesting could eventually lead to extinction. There would be ripple effects considering the fragile nature of ecosystems. One plant might seem insignificant. However, one plant might be everything for so many other plants and animals.

However, scientists that encourage foraging do not see it as a problem. In their opinion, humans would always find a way to protect their survival. That is, if humans decided to eat wild varieties, they would find a way to make them available forever.

Even then, that removes the idea of 'natural' from foraging. Moreover, some species (particularly mushrooms) are not cultivatable. The question is, how do we replace such species?

2. Endangerment of Species

Accidents happen all the time. As humans, no matter how careful we are, we still make mistakes. The severity of these mistakes usually differ. In foraging, even the tiniest mistakes might pose significant risks.

Little mistakes can have grievous effects like stepping on a harmless plant without even knowing. You can find out in the end that those plants are endangered. Also, given the most care, the protection of these endangered species depends on the experience of the forager.

Veterans would quickly know what to avoid and where to avoid them. Beginners, on the other hand, might not find it easy. When brought to entirely new areas, veterans could even make those mistakes.

Sometimes, the excitement that comes with foraging gets the better of some people. You find some individuals doing extra to get some species.

Some of these people find their motivation in the exorbitant prices of these wild plants. Others are just fascinated by their taste. Either way, you see them throwing caution to the wind in satisfying their cravings.

It results in trampling on endangered species. Some could even destroy tree branches to have portions in some wild fruits.

3. Destruction of Natural Ecosystems

Foraging comes with the interference of man with natural environments. Though some might argue that this interference is minimal, even in little amounts, man's intervention could tip the balance of the ecosystems.

This interference could be as small as creating footpaths. No matter how little, man contributes a sort of imbalance to these natural habitats. These slight imbalances in the end aggregate into the extinction of some species.

Encouraging foraging would imply bringing a lot of humans into the wild. Such an influx would undoubtedly disrupt the fragile balance of these habitats.

At the moment, it is estimated that over 12 species go extinct every day. At that rate, if we all decided to forage, it would only be a moment before there's nothing left.

4. Toxicity

One of the significant risks that come with foraging is toxicity. There are so many edible species out there. At the same time, several species are dangerous to consume.

Some of these edibles look so alike with their dangerous counterparts. Sometimes, the best way to tell them apart is by experience. Even with experience, veterans still find it difficult to tell the difference between some plants.

If ingested, toxic plants could cause poisoning. Some others can also cause severe skin irritations for people with allergies.

Final Words

There is no doubt that foraging is beneficial. There are several benefits for humans and the environment at large. However, the benefits of foraging depend on reasonable use. Reasonable use is also a factor of the forager, the land, and several other variables.

Foraging can become a problem, if uncontrolled. Even with the issues that come with unreasonable use, foraging is still beneficial. One of the ways that you can avoid making foraging a problem is using the right tools.

In the next chapter, you will learn all the essential tools you need to get before you go foraging.

Chapter 10

Essential Tools for Foraging

oraging is one of the most frugal and healthiest hobbies you can find. It is a great way to reconnect with nature. It is also an excellent way to explore the outdoors.

For some, foraging is a way of life. Having the right tools will make foraging fun, safe, and a lot easier for you.

15 Essential Tools for Foraging

Having the right tools makes life easier. If you want to go into foraging, some essential tools will make your foraging experience fun.

These tools make foraging easier and enjoyable for you. Though you can do without some of them, there are some you cannot do without.

1. Pruners

Pruning knife is one tool you might not be able to do without as a forager. If it is only one tool you can purchase to get started, pruners are the tool of choice. A pruning knife is useful for cutting vines and stalks.

Pruners are built for this purpose, and its hook-shaped design makes it possible to slice with a single stroke. Also, a dedicated knife helps in mixed terrain, and for cutting low to the ground. You get to protect your survival knife from rust and accidental rock strike.

However, purchasing the right type of pruning knife is essential. Purchase a high-quality pruner that can be sharpened. This quality ensures you don't always have to replace your pruner once it gets blunt.

If possible, purchase a pruner that can be modified with stippling or one with a non-slip handle. This characteristic ensures that it does not slip and cut you.

Purchase a pruner that will reduce strain and hand fatigue. When fully opened, the pruners should not exceed the width of your grasp.

Pruners are used mostly when gathering and processing foraged herbs. They easily snip right through twigs, small branches, roots, and herbaceous stems.

2. Japanese Garden Knife or Weeding Knife

This tool is also known as Hori Hori. Hori Hori is a famous garden knife that originated from Japan. This origin explains why it is called a Japanese knife. The blade is lightweight and ergonomic. It is also one of the essential tools for foragers. It is lightweight and can easily fit into your backpack.

This tool is compact and used for heavy-duty work. It is an excellent weeding tool and a sturdy wildcrafting tool. It helps to break up soil and dig roots from the earth. Garden knives can pry rocks out of the ground and can even cut through most clay soils. It can also be used for dividing roots, cutting sod, and transplanting.

When purchasing a garden knife, you should buy one with a wooden handle as they tend to be stronger than the plastic. Also, purchase one that has a lip at the base of the blade. It will protect your hand if the knife slips.

3. Digging Fork

Digging fork is the tool of choice for digging roots. The tines of the fork can effectively loosen soils and lift branch roots from the earth. Digging forks are less likely to damage roots than a spade or shovel.

Digging fork can also be used in the garden to loosen soil, harvest medicinal roots, and weed. Unlike hay or manure forks that have flat and bendable tines, digging forks have square and sturdy tines.

4. Shovel

There is a high chance you already have this tool hanging out in your garden shed or garage. However, having a couple of different types can be useful. Shovels vary in sizes.

A larger and more easily manipulated shovel is appropriate for you if you do a lot of foraging. You can also stick with the compact version depending on the amount of foraging you do.

A compact shovel is primarily used in foraging to start the removing/harvesting process of tap-rooted plants such as burdock. It is also useful for digging in heavily compacted soils.

Shovels should be well suited for the environment where your intended harvest can be found. Small digging spades will work fine in soft soil, but they are not appropriate for use in an environment with rocky soil.

5. Kitchen Scissors or Shears

You might be wondering why you need kitchen scissors when you already have a knife. Well, you can do without kitchen scissors if you already have a knife.

However, you should also bear in mind that a lot of things are easier done with scissors than with a knife. It also does not cancel the need for a knife as some tasks are better done with a knife.

In essence, they both have different purposes they are well suited for. So, having them both as your foraging tool will make foraging easier for you.

Kitchen scissors are useful for collecting tender-stemmed greens like violet, chickweed, and cleavers. Using a pruning knife for this task can make a muck of the job as pruners are suited for sturdier stems.

Scissors are also better than pruners for stalked plants like Japanese knotweed, burdock, and thistles.

When purchasing your kitchen scissors, keep your eye out for a quality pair that can cut through small branches.

6. Trowel

A trowel is a small hand tool that is used for digging, smoothing, applying, or moving small amounts of particulate or viscous materials. You might not need a trowel depending on the type of foraging you are into.

However, if you need to harvest any roots like burdock, groundnuts, wild carrot, and so on, then you will need a trowel. You are going to need an excellent way to dig these roots up, and trowel is the best tool for this job.

You should only carry the trowel when it is the season for roots to reduce the weight of your backpack.

7. Pocket Knife

A pocket knife comes in handy when you have to peel the bark of medicinal trees, cut mushrooms off wood, or to cut through thick stems. Using a pocket knife reduces the chance of injuring yourself.

8. Baskets with Handle

Baskets will reward you in many ways. They are handy for gathering and drying herbs. Baskets are a must-have for mushroom enthusiasts.

Mushrooms squish easily, and the safest way to store them and keep them intact is to lay them flat in the bottom of a large basket. For convenience, purchase a basket with handles.

Besides, wild herbs, smaller plants, and edible flowers are better kept in a basket, where they are at lower risk of bruising or crushing.

9. Backpack

A quality backpack is one of the essential foraging tools. It is the easiest way to carry your other foraging tools, as well as your finds.

A good backpack should be ideally padded with comfortable straps, and should also be a good size for your body. Lots of pouches and pockets are also a plus as it makes organization easier.

10. Breathable Bags

At harvesting, you need a viable means of carrying the plants you find. If you transport the plants in plastic bags that do not allow for any airflow, the vibrant green leaves might turn brown. The best way to carry these plants is with a breathable container.

You might also need to factor in small containers for berries, mushrooms, and fruits. Certain mushrooms, berries, and soft fruits are fragile. They can be easily crushed in a backpack or even in a foraging basket that is loaded.

Putting them in small containers before keeping them in the backpack or basket will help protect your delicate harvest.

11. Buckets or Tubtrugs

As you become proficient with foraging, you will need buckets for larger-scale harvests such as wild blueberry and elderberry, as well as for muddy root harvests. Adding a little water in the bottom of the buckets will also help to keep the leaves and stems of your herbs fresh throughout the long car ride back home.

12. Gloves

Foraging can be hard on your hands. Plants like nettles or a berry bramble can prick your fingers. If you have ever encountered the stinging sensation from brushing your hand against the fine hairs of nettles, then you know gloves are essential when dealing with plants.

Using gloves will protect your hands and fingertips from pricks. Protect your hands with suitable leather gloves.

13. Magnifying Glass or Loupe

A magnifying lens makes it much easier to spy on flowers.

You will need to look at every detail like the minute pore size, or almost invisible hairs on the plant stems, or small veins in leaves to correctly identify some plants and mushrooms. These details cannot be easily seen just with your eyes. You need a magnifying lens.

14. Clear Glass Plate

You will need a transparent glass plate for spore prints. Making spore prints is crucial for distinguishing the edible mushrooms from poisonous or potentially deadly ones. Spore prints can be made using a transparent glass plate.

15. Water Bottle

Foraging can be dehydrating. You will need a lot of water to keep you going. Therefore, a water bottle is an essential foraging tool.

When purchasing water bottles for foraging, buy a big container that can hold large quantities of water. You should also purchase one that will fit appropriately into your backpack.

Now, you have a checklist of all the tools you need before you go out to forage. However, before you go, you wonder if you can have someone with you. Well, you might not have heard of foraging societies. You can know more about them in the next chapter.

Chapter 11

Foraging Societies:
What You Need to Know

D id you ever play this game where you were lost in the wild and had to look for food for yourself when you were young? You would probably eat the fruits in your garden, pretend to live in a house made from wood, and hunt animals down.

What you probably didn't know then was that it was the way of life of some people. These people are foragers. Yes, there are still people who live that way.

You might wonder how this lifestyle can be sustainable in the 21st century. From previous chapters, you have learned about the benefits of foraging, so you should be able to see why people might want to live this way.

However, you might not have a real idea of how a foraging society is structured, the culture of these people called hunters-gatherers, and the different types of communities. This chapter will help you know all that you need to know.

General Attributes of Foraging Societies

Foraging Societies consist of people who have no consistent source of food. They hunt and gather food, thus the name hunters-gatherers.

These people live a nomadic lifestyle of moving from place to place in search of food. They are also usually small groups to ensure that the food always reaches everyone.

Anthropologists have taken the time to study these societies. You should note that foraging societies are generally hard to consider as a whole due to the different climates where they live. The resources available to the communities also differ, which leads to an inevitable variance in culture.

However, some characteristics are common to all foraging societies. We have discussed a few of them below.

• *Small-Sized Communities*

Foraging Societies are usually small. They also live in places where there are not many people. According to anthropologists, this characteristic is probably so to ensure that the available food will be able to sustain everyone. If they stay in a densely populated area, there is a chance that feeding will become a struggle for survival.

• *Nomadic Lifestyle*

Hunters-Gatherers usually live as nomads. Though it is not the case for all foraging societies, it is common. They only build temporary shelters and move to other areas when there is a need for more food and water. They move with the seasons, herds, and available resources. An example of such a society is the Ngatatjara in the Australian desert.

• Self-Made Tools

Foragers make their tools from materials around in the area. Though, with the increasing development and contact with other communities, they have started making use of machine-made tools.

• Temporal Use of Resources

Foraging societies always make use of available resources in a way that they can regenerate. For instance, they wouldn't uproot fruit-bearing trees, but rather gather the fruits and leave the tree to fruit another year. Once the resources in an area get to a certain level, the foragers move to another area and revisit the area the next season.

• Division of Labor

In foraging societies, everyone works, regardless of gender. The work is usually divided according to gender and age. In King San society of the Kalahari Desert, the women gathered food, which consisted of fruits, melons, berries, and nuts. At the same time, the men performed rituals and entertained the people. In some other societies, the men would hunt, and the females gather vegetation.

• Lack of Structure

Unlike Western societies with their structured political and economic systems, foraging societies do not have such structures in place. These people are often related, and food is commonly shared. They also don't own properties, which can lead to a hierarchy. This lack of a system works since the groups are usually small and related, in addition to the fact that they don't stay in one place.

The way of life in foraging societies is simple and generally alike. The significant differences are in the resources available to them. You can, however, still classify foraging societies based on this factor. You can know the types of foraging groups below.

Types of Foraging Societies

There are traditional features that you can expect to see in any foraging society. However, there are peculiarities by which we can group these societies. Some of the different foraging societies are;

• *Pedestrian Societies*

These societies collect their food while walking around. One well-known foraging society that falls into this category is the Kung San, known as Zhuloasi. This group has access to over 150 species of plants and 100 species of animals.

Zhoulasi does not eat all the plants, though. Their favorite is the mongongo nut, which is a source of protein. They move out of the area once the resources get low or based on the seasons. They live in groups of two or three families in the rainy season but camp out in their twenties or forties when it is dry in a place where there is water.

• *Aquatic Societies*

These foraging societies rely on water to get resources and food for feeding. An example is the Haida, also known as Ou Haadas, who lives in Prince of Wales Island and the Queen Charlotte Islands, British Columbia.

This group uses various kinds of food gotten from the water around their dwellings. Their diet consists of scallops, halibut, otters, salmon, sea lion, and seaweed. However, it is not only what is gotten from the water that they eat.

They also hunt land mammals like deer and gather wild plants like berries.

• *Equestrian Societies*

This group of foragers is rarer than the other two. They identify with only the pampas and steppes of South America and the Great Plains of North America. These types of foragers started after Americans got reintroduced to horses by European settlers.

Aonikenks is an example of this type of foraging society. This society, known as People of the South or Tehuelche, stay on the Patagonian Steppes of South America. They hunt guanaco and eat roots, rhea, and seeds.

Why Foraging Societies are Not Common Anymore

Foraging Societies were the norm for over one million years. However, it is not a lifestyle that you see anymore. You might wonder why it is so.

Well, the change started with the Neolithic Revolution.

About 12,000 years ago, when the Neolithic Revolution began, agriculture started. People had to build houses so they could stay in one place to look after their farms. While hunters-gatherers still existed until the modern age, the lifestyle dwindled until it seems inexistent.

One of the reasons this way of life is uncommon is because of the risks that come with it. There is the possibility of not finding food for days, health risks, and whatnot.

Many people are considering merging this way of life with their current lifestyle, due to the benefits of foraging.

If you had taken the time to read this book to this point, you must be considering some foraging yourself. We congratulate you on that step and hope we have been able to help you on your journey.

Conclusion

Do you remember Bob? Yes, that man that could fend for himself in the wild.

You probably thought that what he did was not attainable when you read his story in the introduction.

However, now that you have gotten to the end of this book, we hope you know differently. You have all it takes to go foraging, and with the help of this book, you won't get it wrong.

Every word in this book has guided you into knowing how to identify and locate regional edible wild plants and mushrooms.

Are you trying to refresh the knowledge you have in your arsenal now? Let's highlight what you got from this book.

You have learned what foraging is, its categories, and commonly asked questions. There is probably no issue about foraging that you cannot tackle now.

Mushrooms are an interesting specie. Now, you know all about their history and how there are edible and non-edible types. Every detail you need to examine to identify, locate, and cultivate the edible species has been highlighted in an easy to read format.

We understood that gathering these edible mushrooms is not the end of the journey. Therefore, you were able to learn all the strategies that you can use to harvest and store mushrooms. These tips will help you enjoy the sweet delicacy of mushrooms for a long time.

As delicious as mushrooms can be, it can get old if it is always a part of your meal without any varieties. Therefore, you need to know how to use, identify, and locate other edible wild plants.

With fifty edible wild plants described and explained in this book, this need should not be a problem at all. You should also know the right methods to use when harvesting and soring these plants.

Foraging comes with its risks and benefits. This book has outlined them for you so that you know what you are doing before you start. We didn't live you without hope, though, as we explained safety tips that will aid you when you are out in the wild.

One of the essential things you need to get right, especially if you are a beginner, is the tools you need for foraging. You now know the fifteen crucial tools that you need to have when you go foraging.

Expert foragers will probably tell you that one of the joys of foraging is the beauty of doing it with friends and family. You have learned about foraging societies, their characteristics, and types.

Can you see that you have all the knowledge you need to start foraging? You would have zero problems identifying, locating, and preserving edible wild plants and mushrooms in your region with this book as your guide.

So, what are you waiting for?

It is time to start foraging!

www.ingramcontent.com/pod-product-compliance
Lightning Source LLC
Chambersburg PA
CBHW062136020426
42335CB00013B/1232